Fit to Fish
How to Tackle Angling Injuries

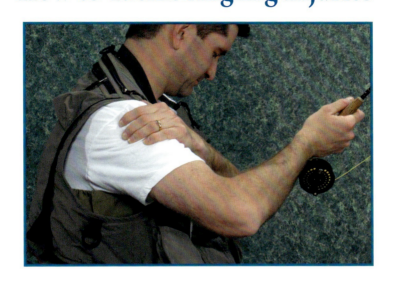

Stephen L. Hisey, P.T.
Keith R. Berend, M.D.

Edited by Barbara Hanno
Illustrations by Julie A. Hisey, PT

Frank Amato

PORTLAND

Dedication

I would like to dedicate this book to God and his many blessings in my life including my wife Julie, and son Ben. They provided ceaseless encouragement and support during this entire project without which I could not have completed the task.

—Steve Hisey P.T.

In loving memory of my mom, Emily Seymour Berend, who first taught me to fish with a cane pole and worms. Whether deep-sea fishing for sailfish off Key Largo, stalking bones on the flats, or drifting dries on the Little Manistee, ready to bait a hook or remove a fish, my mom was the true angler.

—Dr. Keith Berend, M.D.

All inquiries should be addressed to:

Frank Amato Publications, Inc.
P.O. Box 82112, Portland, Oregon 97282
503•653•8108 • www.amatobooks.com

All photographs by the authors except BodyBlade® photos courtesy of BodyBlade®.
Illustrations by Julie A. Hisey, P.T.
Book & Cover Design: Kathy Johnson
Printed in Hong Kong

Softbound ISBN: 1-57188-354-1   UPC: 0-81127-00188-0
1 3 5 7 9 10 8 6 4 2

Contents

About the Authors

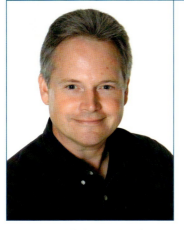

Steve Hisey, P.T.

Steve is a graduate of the University of Washington and completed his BS degree in Physical Therapy in 1981. He began his career working at Evergreen Hospital in Kirkland where he was destined to meet his wife Julie, who at that time was learning the ropes in physical therapy as a student at the University of Washington. Steve enhanced his therapy knowledge treating a broad range of injuries while working for a private practice and then a spine rehabilitation clinic in the Seattle area. Bozeman, Montana lured Steve and his family in 1992 with the promise of less traffic, clean air, and abundant fishing opportunities. After ten years at Advanced Performance and Rehabilitation Services in Bozeman, Steve ventured into practice with his wife at her established practice, Bozeman Manual Therapy. Steve continues to expand his working knowledge of therapy and fishing through on-stream "research" in surrounding rivers, lakes, and streams.

Keith R. Berend, M.D.

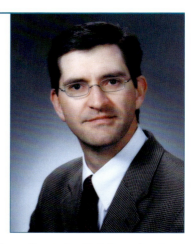

A native of Columbus, Ohio, I spent every summer of my life on the shore of Lake Michigan with my mom, dad, and grandfather, many a morning spent trolling for salmon or fly-fishing the Little Manistee. I learned to fly-fish with my grandfather at age 5 with a 9-foot fiberglass fly rod and empty hooks. The rod is now about 3 feet shorter, but still functional in the hands of my daughters (Taylor age 7, and Molly age 5). After graduating high school in Columbus, warmer climates were in sight at Florida Southern College in Lakeland, Florida. From there it was Duke University for Medical School and Orthopedic Surgery residency training. It was in Durham that I first got the itch to write about fishing. In *North Carolina Wildlife* magazine, my first feature article was about float tube fly-fishing the many farm ponds around the city. Duke was also the starting ground for my interest in fly-fishing-related maladies, their treatment and prevention. My family and I spent 6 months in western North Carolina working some, but fishing plenty. This served as the perfect backdrop to introduce my wife, Cindy, to the sport. I have now returned to Columbus, where I practice Orthopedic Surgery with a specialty interest in hip and knee replacements. We visit Michigan to fish the Pere Marquette, the Au Sable, and the Little Manistee as often as time allows, and still love trolling for big salmon as well. My addiction, fortunately or unfortunately, has also led to a passion for flats-fishing and offshore fly-fishing in the Florida Keys where we spend time with my number-one fishing partner, my dad, John Berend.

Foreword

I first bumped into Steve at a Trout Unlimited meeting in Bozeman several years ago while giving a casting instruction seminar highlighting some useful casting techniques that I have used over the years. My 35 years of experience teaching fly-casting, guiding and running a fly-fishing shop in West Yellowstone has exposed me to all sorts of useful casting tips that solve a variety of problems encountered while plying the waters for fish. Over the years it has been my privilege to have worked and taught fly-casting with and learned from some of the finest fly-casting instructors in the world. People like Lefty Kreh, Joan and Lee Wulff, Mel Krieger, Gary Borger and many others. Trout that are surface feeding in flat water may require a straight downstream or a down-and-across presentation and approach. Throwing a bounce cast/checking the cast straight down stream lands the fly in front of its prey with plenty of slack in the leader and tippet to prevent drag. The fly is the first thing that comes into view making for an appetizing presentation for the unsuspecting fish. Problem solved.

This book takes a similar approach and applies it to problems encountered in the fisherman's body. Steve Hisey and Dr. Keith Berend have observed the many aches and pains we encounter on stream and have come up with solutions to these problems by applying their knowledge of medicine and fishing. *Fit to Fish* is the first book of its kind to describe common fishing maladies, explain how they happen, and then give advice on what can be done to correct them. There is plenty of practical information packed in these pages which can go a long way towards making fishing less painful and more productive.

I learned a little human anatomy along the way as it is used throughout the book to illustrate the nature of injuries and how casting can result in overuse injuries of our body parts. Much of the anatomy language has a familiar ring to it because it is based on Latin which is the same language used to define insects and their life cycles. Just as understanding the details of aquatic insect life is helpful in catching trout, knowledge of human anatomy enables better performance of the amazing machine we live in.

Latin, or no Latin, there are plenty of useful stretching and strengthening exercises described in this book which can be applied to the arms, trunk, or legs without any in-depth knowledge of anatomy. It's kind of like an owner's manual for fishermen where you can choose to flip to any chapter in the book and read up on the specific joint you have questions about.

This book got me thinking about changes I can make to improve my fishing experience with regards to better physical comfort, improved casting performance, and injury prevention. It's definitely worth the read and to have in one's library for future reference and help.

—*Bob Jacklin*
December 12, 2004

Introduction

There remains considerable debate as to the actual origin of fly-fishing. Some believe the sport existed as far back as A.D. 1200 while others argue that fly-fishing did not arise until famous books and treatises on the subject surfaced from the 1400's through the 1800's. Still others argue the burgeoning interest in fly-fishing should be credited to Robert Redford and Brad Pitt. In the classic book and feature movie, *A River Runs Through It*, Norman MacLean states: "Something within fishermen tries to make fishing into a world perfect and apart—I don't know what it is or where, because sometimes it is in my arms and sometimes in my throat and sometimes nowhere in particular except somewhere deep."

We are not vain enough to believe that Norman was alluding to arm pain, neck discomforts, or that "somewhere deep" was the lower lumbar spine, but it is intriguing to wonder if Paul, Norman, or Reverend MacLean had shoulder bursitis, elbow tendonitis, or low back pain. A s an orthopedic surgeon and physical therapist, we are challenged daily with diagnosing, treating, and preventing the common musculoskeletal problems from which people suffer. Whether patients swing golf clubs, stroke tennis balls, jog trails, or just lounge around; they have specific complaints that need to be addressed. Just as specific ailments are associated with golf, tennis, and running, fly-fishing too has its own set of physical maladies. Those maladies associated with our sport of repetitively beating the water with the long rod, are addressed in this text. We deal with fly-fishing and its assault on our musculoskeletal system, as well as those methods that can be employed to lessen the toll. We provide an overview of common disorders prevalent in fly anglers, explain the causes, and describe treatment and prevention techniques utilizing conditioning, stretching, and exercise. So join us in this mission to bring fly-fishing to the foreground as a true sport, with triumph and defeat, with wholeness and injury, and with joy and pain.

"If there is pleasure, then pain will follow": This is not a direct quote from the IRS tax code manual, but with over seventy-five years of combined experience treating the human body, we have verified this basic concept many times over. A way to restate this is, "If it feels good today, it will probably hurt tomorrow." Life in abundance extracts a certain price from the mass of cells in which we live, whether it's done suddenly without warning, or in a seductively slow fashion. We cannot escape this fundamental truth.

> *Life in abundance extracts a certain price from the mass of cells in which we live, whether it's done suddenly without warning, or in a seductively slow fashion.*

Given the inevitable nature of pleasure and resulting pain, it only seems appropriate to find ways to minimize the damage and speed the healing. This writing is an attempt to address fly-fishing and its assault on our musculoskeletal system as well as those methods which can be employed to lessen the toll. Three sources of experience have contributed to our overall understanding of pain. First and foremost is our day-to-day floundering through life's classrooms of trial and error. Although this did not produce a diploma, it nevertheless played a major role in establishing a need for this book. Secondly, our perspectives as a physical therapist and an orthopedic surgeon have formalized our understanding of pain. Last, but not least, is our understanding of fishing, especially fly-fishing, as a major source of pleasure. These three areas of experience provide us with a practical approach in dealing with unpleasant ailments that prevent or diminish the fly-fishing experience.

A clinical research study examined the maladies and aliments that plague many of us who spend time on the water.[1] The results of this study, the first of its kind, have opened the eyes of the flyfishing world to the real nature of our pains that relate to fly-fishing. It is on this backbone that this book is written.

We did not explore all acute traumatic injuries and their first aid. This has been covered elsewhere. Rather, we focused primarily on overuse injuries that we have experienced as anglers or treated in our professions as therapist and surgeon. At the very least, these injuries nag us as we pursue our most pleasant addiction. Left untreated, they have the potential to completely destroy our ability and desire to fish. We hope that fish slime and scales will eventually adorn the pages of this book so that needless suffering is avoided and fishing time is extended.

1. Prevalence of Orthopaedic Maladies in People Who Flyfish: An Internet-Based Survey, Keith R. Berend, MD: Journal of the Southern Orthopedic Association 10:221-220, 2001

1
CHAPTER

Fishing and Pain

Fishing and Pain: The Therapist's Story

I had pulled ashore at the lower end of a pool so clear and smooth it has earned the name "The Aquarium". *Trico* spinners littered the surface film and appeared to transport over rising browns like a sheet-glass conveyer belt. A steady rolling motion exposing only dorsal fins summoned me into deceptively waist-deep water. Strong similarity existed between this scene and one I had observed years ago while waiting to wind surf a gusty day on Puget Sound. These were not the killer whales I had seen there, however, their steady, rhythmical, and rolling motion in a close "pod" suggested a similar ancestry and feeding behavior.

Six X and a size-twenty Trico spinner were the order of the day. Adrenaline in saturation nearly destroyed my ability to link fly and line. Staring intensely at my shaking fingers, working tippet to hook became more difficult when sounds of the pod feeding reached my ears. This new course of chemically induced excitement felt good as it always had, despite its negative effects on my dexterity.

Fear of shattering a delicate feeding frenzy kept my wading to no closer than thirty feet. Casts down and across also aided in landing the decoy undetected by its prey. Slowly my attempts landed closer to the actual feeding lane inhabited by the pod. At that point it was a simple game of numbers as my fly was on course, conveyed over the line of rolling fish at the same speed and direction as the rest of their meal. Sunshine warmed morning fingers to life, but also added to the difficult viewing of my fly sitting flat on the surface. As in reading the smallest letters on an eye exam, I naturally leaned forward, jutting my head out in attempts at getting a closer look at my tiny fly. Despite the impossibility of visualizing my creation, I persisted with this technique for some time as adrenaline dictated the importance of seeing the first strike. Repeated floats through the gauntlet did nothing but instill more of the same behavior in the pod, and it was painfully obvious that these fish were happily devouring cheap imitations of my fly that were all around.

Time began to warp as it usually does while in pursuit of a trophy on the river. The sudden surprise of a seventeen-inch brown launching itself in the middle of the pod caught my attention, as did the realization that he was somehow magically attached to my rod. Instincts quickly overcame my slow processing of what had just occurred, resulting in a successful landing of my first fish.

Upon release of this first "whale" I was allowed to interpret sensory input from all parts of my body again: cold feet, tired wrists, slimy fingers, and *pain* in my neck. Where did the neck pain come from? All other sensations were expected, but the neck pain was new and troublesome. Stiffness with motion and a nagging ache at the base of my neck did not fit with the other senses usually encountered while wading. The joy of catching my first fish of the fall season using a size-20 dry fly gave me sudden insight into the cause.

Most, if not all, of my previous fishing that year involved nymphing at close range with a buoyant and bright strike indicator. Dry-fly-fishing earlier that year employed larger and more visible patterns, ensuring little eyestrain. This neck pain was the direct result of poor posture for a prolonged period of time. Straining to see my *Trico* under the influence of intoxicating circumstances for several hours, caused a forward jutting of my head and neck, resulting in irritation to the spine and supporting muscles. I have since experienced the same type of pain and usually associate it with fishing small dries at distance. Adding to this postural strain at the neck is the frequent false casting that is required to re-float a dry repeatedly all day.

Not all pain comes from acute injury as this episode illustrates. Many afflictions are brought on by poor posture or overuse of a particular body part for a prolonged time. The majority of this type of pain that is produced while fishing can gradually get worse the more the given area is used, or used incorrectly. Changing posture or fishing technique is usually a major part of getting well. Sudden increases in the amount a body part is used will overtax the area if it is not conditioned for the loads applied. Early spring fishing can be one of the most vulnerable times of the year for overuse injuries as you move from the tying bench to the rivers and begin using body parts unchallenged all winter.

Trauma, i.e., falling on your *keister,* can produce lingering pain that affects fishing quality. Many of these strains, sprains, and bruises initiate chronic tendonitis or bursitis if left untreated. Not as common in fishing, due to the basic non-contact nature of the sport, traumatic injuries still present a major hurdle to fishing comfortably. We included traumatic injuries acquired during fishing that may also be aggravated by fishing.

Environmental conditions that may promote pain are usually present while wading. One quality of water is its ability to lubricate a surface, making clinging to it difficult or even impossible. How many slippery rocks, boat floors, and wet grass banks have you slid on? My greatest concern when getting out of my friend's aluminum drift boat is firm footing as I step over the rather high gunwale. I still have an exquisite pain memory of a day on the Madison River in Montana. As I stepped out of the boat with one leg, the foot still in the boat slipped, resulting in a two-point landing directly centered on the gunwale! No physical therapy in the world can ease that pain. Although not a common injury, this is one example of water and its deleterious effects on the surfaces we fish on.

Not to be outdone by water is its close relative, ice. I enjoy winter fishing whenever the temperature hovers briefly above 33 degrees, allowing several casts before the rod guides freeze to the line and need cleaning. The usual solitude of winter fishing enhances the experience and can lead to a great day of fishing the midday midge hatch. However, covering vast stretches of ice-covered, freestone banks is a major concern lest you fall and break an ankle. No need to rewrite one of your own chapters of *To Build A Fire*.

Many injuries arise from the very slippery conditions created by Mother Nature to cradle our favorite prey. Along with the need for a water environment, fish generally need cold water (relative to us) to thrive. We include this environmental condition, because it has a substantial impact on how the body functions. Cold water or air increases the stiffness felt in any injured or arthritic joint, making it a challenge to use after several hours in waist-deep water. Prime trout water is in the range of 55 to 65 degrees, which is substantially lower than our own 98.6 core body temperature. Even with recent wader technology, it is difficult to keep your legs and feet above the stream temperature for more than a few hours. Meantime, cold air can wreak havoc with the exposed fingers and neck, making even the simplest movements agonizing. The best solutions are to cover your exposed body parts and make frequent trips to the bank for a fast warm-up walk. Cold can create new injuries or irritate old ones even when prevention and caution are used.

Overuse or traumatic injury brings out the worst in your body and prevents you from pursuing happiness. Environmental conditions add to these aches and pains and multiply their effect on your physical dysfunction. Understanding pain and its origins will enable you to delay or reduce the effects of injury as you participate in your favorite sport.

Fishing and Pain: A Surgeon's Tale

During my medical training, I had the opportunity to spend a lengthy tour of duty at the Veteran's Hospital in Asheville, North Carolina, serving those who served our country. Between the government schedule and the long summer days, I was able to pursue the tight line on many occasions. Through a friend, I gained access to some extremely well-managed private water in the Smoky Mountains, where a riffle ran into a huge pool we named Jurassic Park. After almost a decade of meticulous management, the fish in the pool were of enormous size and tremendous stature. Late one evening, my closest fishing ally and I were hunched behind a large boulder, taking turns throwing dry flies at willing brown and orange beasts. When I turned to see how John was doing with his quarry, I found he had taken a respite on a nearby hammock. I, of course, prodded and teased that he was much less the angler than I, but he said his back hurt and he had shooting pains in the groin and anterior thigh. Well, several releases and many exaggerated stories later, we discovered that John had arthritis in his back. The only thing that caused him discomfort was the posture required by stealthy approach to the pool, the swift current, and the unsteady footing of the streambed. He could plow a field, haul loads of dirt and rock, a real tractor of a man, but fly-fishing caused him severe discomfort that required him to lie down often just to find relief.

Not a week later, I found myself dispensing tales of tails and sharing coffee at the local fly shop when not one, but two, friends entered the store—one adorned with an elbow brace and the other clad in a wrist brace. Both complained that they had aggravated "that old injury" during a recent trip to the coast in pursuit of false albacore. I couldn't believe it. Three fly-fishermen, three ailments. Not all were directly caused by fishing, but all three were exacerbated by it. All three appeared to be the rate limited step in the equation: fly-fishing plus free time equals tremendous fun.

> *I couldn't believe it. Three fly-fishermen, three ailments. Not all were directly caused by fishing, but all three were exacerbated by it.*

That is when I decided to investigate this phenomenon further. Using the scientific method to seek the truth about fishing and pain, I designed, implemented, and published an Internet-based survey study on the orthopedic maladies in people who fly-fish. Throughout this book, with the help of a licensed physical therapist, we have pulled the information from that study and tied it to proven therapies for those ailments.

2

Pain and Its Origins

Denial

Traumatic or overuse injuries have the potential to cut short any fishing adventure if dealt with in the usual manner—DENIAL. All humans prove extremely capable when it comes to avoiding problems by simply turning the cheek and ignoring them as they are encountered. This technique usually comes back to nail you when dealing with pain. Pain is one method your body has to communicate its current status, and requires a listening brain if it's to be heard. Unfortunately, many aches and pains are mild and intermittent in nature and are easily ignored or hung up on when the signal is sent to the brain. I suppose this may come in handy when pulling a barbed hook from your lip, however, it can lead to more serious injury when dealing with chronic pain. A very simple premise learned over the years is that the earlier an injury can be dealt with, the faster and more completely it can be treated. Repeated grinding on the rotator cuff tendons due to chronic impingement syndrome of the shoulder creates more scar tissue than can be fully resolved. Surgery may regain seventy to eighty percent of the original function, making surgery a last resort. Pay attention or pay the price!

Once we acknowledge that something is wrong, we're half way home. Pain can be thought of as our body's sixth sense. It is a wake-up call, alerting the brain of potential harm. A rare genetic condition exists, known as Riley-Day Syndrome, in which humans are born with the inability to perceive pain at the brain level. Testing has shown that painful stimulus may indeed be "felt" by the affected subject, but their brain is unable to attach the usual discomfort normally associated with the stimulus. These individuals frequently die at an early age as they are constantly at a high risk of serious injury. Thank God for pain!

Pain Sensors

Most structures of the body are loaded with nerve endings, sitting idle and patiently waiting to detect early problems that arise at a cellular level. More of our cars are now equipped with this delicate and precise feature, allowing us to avoid serious breakdowns before they happen! If I had this diagnostic feature in my Subaru, I may have been able to avoid that embarrassing breakdown last summer at 6:30 A.M. when my timing belt broke while traveling in Montana between Hardin and Fort Smith. Thank God for cellular phones and AAA. Anyway, the body has amazing powers to detect problems early before major damage occurs. Our job is to listen and react!

Nerve endings have been cleverly designed by the Creator to detect a variety of problems, including chemical inflammation, tissue tearing, postural pain, and even broken bones. Several types of sensory nerve endings are designed to detect different types of trouble. Although many of these create a similar perception of pain, they all have slightly different signatures perceived by the brain that the owner can use to sort out what is wrong.

Input from pain sensors can be broken down into two basic categories including mechanical and chemical pain receptors. Most acute traumatic injuries create pain first by physically disrupting nerve endings in soft tissues and sending an immediate and intense message: Severe, sharp pain quickly following injury to superficial structures. Pain that begins several seconds or minutes following an injury and involves throbbing is usually caused by damage to mechanical nerve endings of deeper structures like ligaments and joints. These impulses are transmitted over nerve fibers, which carry the pain message to the brain at a slower speed and are somewhat more vague in nature. You usually know you've done something wrong, but it may be difficult to tell exactly what body part is injured. Mechanical pain increases in intensity when the injured part is stressed, and decreases in intensity when the stress is removed. Walking on a sprained ankle results in a limp every time weight is placed on the injured ankle and stress is applied to the injured ligaments.

Inflammation Pain

Natural agents released from the body during the inflammation response produce chemical pain. This inflammation response is a cascade of chemical events that occurs when soft tissues are injured and the body responds with its "first aid" to begin to heal the area. Unfortunately, part of the response includes release of several chemical substances including prostaglandins, which irritate certain nerve endings and result in production of more pain. This type of chemically induced pain can also occur as a throbbing ache, which begins hours or minutes from the time of initial injury. Inflammation pain tends to be constant all day and may be slightly worse at rest or at night when attempting to sleep. Chronic inflammation may be experienced as a constant burning sensation. Inflammation can be quite deceptive in that it may feel less intense during or immediately after exercise. This "warm-up effect" can mislead the athlete or fisherman into thinking that exercise is helping the problem and that the only rational cure to the problem is to fish longer and harder! Disastrous results begin that night or the next morning when increased inflammation from overworking the area leads to more pain. Not to say that exercise is bad. Exercise plays an important role in the healing process, but needs to be added gradually and in small doses so that excessive inflammation is not evoked.

Not all pain falls neatly in these categories and can be frustrating to diagnose. More often than not, injury or overuse involves a combination of the symptoms described above, because more than one process is occurring. Mechanical pain indicates structural damage to soft tissue, and chemical pain ensues later, due to the inflammation response that is evoked. A combination of the two sources of pain is more common in acute traumatic injuries and should be expected.

Referred Pain

Referral of pain to another uninvolved body part is an important characteristic of pain. It can be extremely misleading. That is, injury to deep structures can create fairly constant and severe pain that shows up quite some distance from the injured part. At the same time, the injured area may be completely pain free. The spine is one of the most common body parts that refer pain to other areas. Low back injury frequently radiates pain into the hips and down the back and sides of the thighs. It is not uncommon that pain from a hip joint injury is present only at the knee joint. Referred pain from the musculoskeletal system usually radiates into body parts that are lower than the affected part. Testing of different structures passively is needed to determine which body part is causing the referred pain. When movement of the low back increases the leg pain, then the back may be responsible for the pain. An evaluation by an experienced physical therapist or orthopedist can be of great value in determining the actual injured structure.

Internal organs are notorious for referring pain into the arms and legs. Heart ailments commonly radiate pain into the arms or neck. Pain that does *not* increase or decrease with change in body position should be suspect. This type of referred visceral pain can also increase in intensity at rest, especially at night when attempting to sleep. Be aware of associated symptoms that may occur along with pain, as these are good indicators of possible internal organ disease or damage. I recently treated a young mother who was sent to our clinic for back pain and possible disc herniation. After a week of treatment and a gradual increase in pain down her leg, I sent her back to her M.D. for further evaluation. She recently called back to inform me that she was finally diagnosed using an ultrasound scan, which demonstrated a Fallopian tube cyst. This was successfully removed surgically, and she is now pain free. When in doubt, check it out!

In summary, there are several types of pain generators throughout the body that respond to both mechanical and chemical irritation. Stimulation of these nerve endings can occur by acute trauma or by overuse. Sorting out the types of pain produced helps identify both the damaged structure and the type of injury sustained. Pain is often referred down from the injured area making initial diagnosis more confusing. Referral from internal organs can also create pain in the legs or arms making diagnosis more challenging. Most importantly, pain is a sense the body employs to direct maintenance to itself. Our job is to listen and respond.

> *Most importantly, pain is a sense the body employs to direct maintenance to itself. Our job is to listen and respond.*

Basic Concepts of Self-Treatment

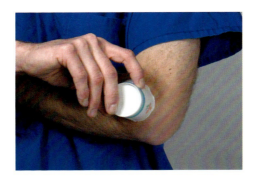

Once we acknowledge pain exists and are willing to deal with it, what's next? Buy a new body and start over. We wish. No, we're pretty much stuck with the original equipment and need to help it heal in order to get on with hunting fish. Healing is one miracle that living organisms perform to themselves, given the opportunity and a little help from the owner. I would have gladly put an ice pack on my Honda Prelude every day and stretched the transmission frequently if I could have avoided having a mechanic rebuild the engine for a mere $2,000. The point is this: A few basic treatment techniques are all that are needed to heal the vast majority of injuries and can easily be self-administered, avoiding needless trips to the doctor or therapist.

First aid

The sooner treatment is given, the less damage occurs and the faster the injured area can be healed and returned to use. Another term for early treatment is first aid. Immediately after any acute injury is the time to begin treatment. Out of sports medicine has come PRICE, an acronym for **P**rotection, **R**est, **I**ce, **C**ompression, **E**levation.

Protection

After spraining a wrist from slipping on a wet rock, it's important to protect the joint from more trauma by bracing the joint. Bracing the injured joint forces that part into temporary retirement and allows other surrounding joints and muscles to take up the slack. Applying a brace over the injured area lessens the workload to that joint, which allows a modified continuation of the same activity to occur more safely. This form of rest is usually recommended in an emergency situation and continues long enough to allow time, therapeutic exercise, and other treatments to heal the injury. An emergency situation (like being injured in the middle of a one-week fly-in Alaskan fishing vacation that costs the angler $4,000) is an appropriate circumstance for the use of a brace to allow continued fishing. Bracing is also routinely used throughout all stages of rehabilitation in order to provide lower levels of loading to the ligaments and tendons while they are gradually healing and adapting to progressively higher loads. Most modern braces provide some compression and proprioceptive feedback to assist in controlling unstable joint motions during activity. Additionally, an arthritic joint may require long-term bracing during activities, due to permanent damage to cartilage that can't be changed with exercise and treatment alone.

Rest

One of the toughest decisions you have to make as an injured athlete/fisherman involves deciding when to take a *rest* from an aggravating activity. Even if you luck out and find a brace in the Alaskan bush for that sprained wrist, you should cut back on the number of hours spent fishing to allow the wrist to heal. Eliminating those midnight fishing hours may be just the ticket to get you through the daylight hours until the end of the week-long trip. Decreasing the use of an injured or inflamed joint results in a faster and more complete recovery, and has the secondary benefit of freeing up time to apply ice and perform beneficial exercises. Used early on, rest is the most beneficial way to reduce pain and restore function, yet is the most ignored rehab aspect, due to the restricted life style and relative boredom that results.

Ice

Soaking the wrist immediately in an *ice* cold stream decreases pain and prevents both severe swelling and inflammation from spreading into other cells that surround the injury. Applying ice or cold for twenty minutes every two hours will do the job. If you don't have an ice-cold stream handy, a bag of frozen peas wrapped in a pillow-case and applied to the area will do the job.

Ice massage is another very effective way to cool a superficial area. This involves freezing water in a paper or Styrofoam cup, then pealing the top down one inch to expose the ice.

Move the exposed ice is in a circular motion over the painful area for eight to ten minutes, producing a red, numb patch of skin over the injured site. Ice massage penetrates more quickly and deeply than an ice pack. The challenge with ice massage is surviving the first three to four minutes of burning and aching until the skin turns red and numb to the touch. Many of my patients express concern for my mental health during the first few minutes of their ice massage as they are worried that I gain too much pleasure from applying it! I always reply with, "just doing my job".

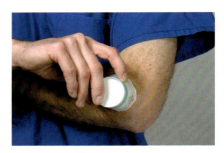

Ice massage.

Keep icing the area repeatedly for several days, or as long as the part hurts at rest. Gradually decrease the frequency of icing to two to three times per day. If there is ever a question about whether using ice or heat is most appropriate, always error by using ice initially, as heat application speeds up the inflammation process and spreads it into surrounding cells, causing more damage. Heat can be beneficial weeks after acute injury, or with arthritis, as it can be applied prior to an exercise session to increase circulation, relax muscles, and improve potential gains in flexibility while stretching. This exercise session should then be followed with ice application to reduce any inflammation that may have resulted.

Compression

Wrapping the wrist with an ace wrap, bandanna, or elastic sleeve will *compress* the area preventing a progression of swelling. Caution! Don't wrap any area too tight, because this may cut off circulation. Tension the ace wrap so you can get two fingers under it easily. Check your fingers or toes on a regular basis to ensure that you have no increased swelling, blue or white coloration, or tingling. These are all signs that the compression wrap is too tight. You will get the most out of compression if it is applied first thing in the morning, taken off and rewrapped at noon, and taken off completely in the evening when you are able to elevate the limb.

Elevation

Give the keys to your friend and let him or her drive you home. Keep the wrist *elevated* above the level of your heart, allowing drainage of swelling from the limb. Keeping a body part above heart level allows gravity to assist in draining fluid out of that limb and minimizes damage to other cells in that area.

This simple group of treatments goes a long way to preventing further cell damage caused by swelling and speeds the healing process. The time frame is critical, meaning the sooner the better. Fishing two more hours and then applying these treatments is worthless. Studies have shown that most cellular damage from swelling occurs in the first few hours after an injury and is as much a cause of cell death as the original trauma! Take the rest of the day off and treat the area, or you could add several weeks or months to the total healing time.

> ### *Take the rest of the day off and treat the area, or you could add several weeks or months to the total healing time.*

Transverse Friction Massage

Once the acute inflammation stage has decreased and the injured area no longer throbs at rest, further treatment methods can be employed to hasten your return to the river. Transverse friction massage is a commonly used technique that can be applied to most tendon and ligament injuries. This technique involves placing the pads of two or three fingers perpendicularly over the sore area, and moving the skin back and forth quickly without letting your fingers slide on the skin.

Friction massage can be applied lightly for two to three minutes over an acutely inflamed tendon, or applied more deeply for ten minutes over an old chronic injury that is less tender to the touch. Vary the time and intensity according to the level of tenderness. Most sore tendons will become "numb" as the massage is applied over the first two to three minutes, keep going! This is a tem-

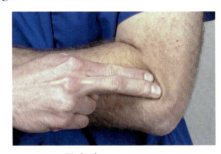

Friction massage.

porary analgesic affect that may last a few hours, and is a good sign that friction massage will be beneficial to healing this particular tendon. Some tendon injuries will not experience this numbing effect during friction massage even after three or four separate sessions of application. In this case, you are probably wise to quit trying friction massage for a few weeks and use other less painful treatments. You will find that you are able to come back to this technique when the tendon is less sore, and achieve better results.

The human body will heal a tendon or ligament by laying down new collagen fibers haphazardly over the injury, resulting in fibers pointing in all directions. This will glue the tear together quickly, but results in a weaker tendon as many of the fibers are not aligned with the orientation of the tendon. In addition, these fibers tend to glue down and attach to other structures in the area, resulting in decreased mobility.

Friction massage has two important mechanical effects when applied correctly. First, rubbing perpendicular to the tendon length, or across the grain, will reorganize new collagen fibers so that they lay down parallel to one another. To illustrate this affect, rub your hand over a pile of pick-up-sticks on a hard floor and observe how they will fall in line parallel to each other. Parallel fibers aligned with the length of the tendon provide for stronger tensile strength. This is analogous to steel cable, which is strong because individual steel wires are combined in a parallel orientation so that each wire is able to resist forces in the same direction.

A second important benefit of friction massage includes the stimulation of blood flow to the area. Just as rubbing your skin turns it red, moving the skin back and forth over the tendon helps to turn it red with fresh blood flow. Improved blood flow results in faster healing by moving nutrients into the cells, while at the same time, flushing waste products out of the cells.

This is a very simple and effective technique that can be self-administered several times per day. Soon, you will find yourself unconsciously rubbing your elbow throughout the day as you discover the addiction to friction.

Posture and Alignment

Postural alignment of the extremities and spine is important for pain-free function, because alignment places your system in a balanced state, reducing stress to joints and soft tissues. Guide wires from all sides can hold tall radio and TV towers erect relatively easily. This is due to the structural balance of each tower segment one on top of the other. If one section of the tower were to be positioned off to one side, every segment above would be positioned off center, causing the entire top portion to lean in that direction. A huge additional tension load would then be placed on the guide wires and connections (muscles, tendons, and ligaments) resulting in immediate breakage or early collapse of that tower (body).

Many injuries cause body parts to be poorly aligned, and many poorly aligned body parts cause injuries. Looking at alignment early in the rehabilitation process is crucial so that balance is achieved and stress to the injured area is decreased. Neck pain due to poor posture is a classic example where the primary cure is simply a postural change. Rebalancing the system removes excess loads from the muscles and joints of the spine and pain is diminished. Similarly, many shoulder joint problems are caused by a weakness in the muscles that support the *scapula* (or shoulder blade) which is the foundation for the shoulder. Weak scapular muscles lead to a forward slumped scapula which places extra loads on the rotator cuff mechanism. And with overuse, this may result in tendon breakdown with subsequent inflammation.

Most alignment problems require several changes for you to notice improvement. Thinking about posture is the first step. A second step involves strengthening supportive muscles that cross the involved joint. The postural change then becomes subconscious and easier to assume and maintain. A final step is stretching tight muscles that restrict proper alignment.

Stretching

Good posture requires a combination of flexibility, strength, and muscle control. Flexibility is the next component of an effective treatment for most injuries. It can only be gained with a nasty practice called "exercise". Although many attempts have been made over the years to substitute technology for exercise, it is still one essential element needed in most rehabilitation programs. Exercise by nature is an active endeavor that requires your involvement. Hi-tech machines have been developed which enhance exercise, but none can replace the active component required by each of us. This is the point at which many rehab programs fail, as our passive nature usually overrides our need for active exercise, and several hours in front of the TV replaces a few minutes with the appropriate exercise.

> *This is the point at which many rehab programs fail, as our passive nature usually overrides our need for active exercise, and several hours in front of the TV replaces a few minutes with the appropriate exercise.*

Maintaining full flexibility is important to maximize function because this determines the range of motion through which a body part is allowed to move. A good golf swing demands excellent trunk and hip mobility so that rotation is driven from the central body core outward to the club. Loss of motion in the trunk causes additional motion in the legs and arms, resulting in a less powerful and less accurate swing. Lost motion in one joint forces more motion to occur in other joints, which can result in injury.

Along with maintaining full motion, stretching decreases stress on your soft tissues by lengthening them and allowing for greater slack in these tissues at rest. Injured soft tissues heal by rebuilding with fibers of the same tissue type (i.e. tendon) as well as with scar tissue fibers blended together. Scar tissue has the property of shrinking into itself slowly over time if not stretched regularly during early healing. A good example of this characteristic can be seen with burn scars. Untreated, they look like a spider with long strands of tissue contracting toward the center of the scar. Frequent stretching and use of elastic pressure garments are the only means of reorganizing burn scars to help prevent the unsightly shrinkage and deformity that would otherwise occur. These techniques are applied as soon as possible following a severe burn, as they are most effective over the first few months while the scar tissue is maturing.

Frequent stretching of an injured tendon elongates it and places it in a slackened position while at rest. Nagging pain at rest can originate from a structure that is too short, and, consequently, exerts a steady stress to the surrounding joint and soft tissues. Every tendon, muscle, and ligament in the body has hundreds of mechanical nerve endings that sense when abnormal loads are placed on them. An easy demonstration of this "mechanical" pain is achieved by grabbing your index finger by the tip and pulling it backward slowly towards the forearm. At a certain point, this stretch loads the tendon significantly, firing nerve endings inside the tendon causing the perception of pain in your finger and palm. An injured tendon or ligament that heals tightly has this same kind of tension on it at rest or with certain postures. Lengthening the tendon by stretching it will turn off the mechanical nerve endings within the tendon and diminish the pain while at rest.

Stretching and strengthening exercises also assist in increasing the strength of tendons and ligaments by applying a load across these structures as they heal. Tendons, muscles, and ligaments are composed of microscopic fibers that are bundled together and are all aligned in the same direction. A piece of steel cable has this similar organization. Repeated stretching and strengthening exercises place an elevated stress across the healing fibers which induce them to become stronger over time.

A research study produced clear electron microscope images that demonstrated physical differences between rabbit tendons that were given exercise while healing versus tendons that were not exercised. Tendons of both groups were initially cut in two and then sutured back together. Those rabbits that were placed in a cast for eight weeks without exercise showed masses of new, frayed fibers lying down in all directions. In contrast, the images of rabbits placed in removable splints and given daily stretching and strengthening exercises showed tendon fibers that were smoother and more parallel to each other. Now, we're not interested in how our tendons look under a microscope, but these differences translate to the strength of the repairs. At the end of the experiment, the tendons were removed from the rabbits and were tested for tensile strength by pulling on each end to the point of rupture. Rabbit tendons that were exercised regularly during their recovery were almost twice as strong as the rabbit tendons that were not given exercise.

Perform each stretching exercise for 30-60 seconds and stop motion at the point of pain if present. Repeat each stretching exercise 3-5 repetitions with a short rest between. Maximum benefit will occur if the stretching exercise sessions are repeated at least 3 times per day.

Strengthening

Muscle is the only tissue in the body that can actively shorten or lengthen itself and exert external motion in the process. Okay, so some humans have the same ability to expand their head size simply by inflating their egos. This is outside the realm of normal physiology and must be considered an exception. Muscles shorten and lengthen at our command. A good false cast requires a symphony of hundreds of muscles firing at the precise time and intensity to accurately guide our fly to the target. Repeating this cast every few minutes over an eight-hour day requires muscles that have both strength and endurance.

Muscle weakness or loss of endurance can cause an overuse injury. A weak rotator cuff or shoulder blade muscle group can produce an overuse injury to the rotator cuff muscles by allowing increased pinching, or impingement, of the rotator cuff tendons during repeated casting. Following injury to the rotator cuff, pain restricts use of the shoulder and results in a gradual weakening of the rotator cuff muscles. This example illustrates the importance of maintaining good muscle strength to prevent injury, as well as allowing healing from an injury. Strengthening exercises are a critical part of any rehabilitation program, but should also be included in any preventive program.

Good muscular strength is beneficial for four reasons: First, strong muscles dynamically support joints in an erect postural alignment, which is ultimately more efficient. If posture were not important for optimum function, you would routinely see competitive athletes standing in a slumped position. When was the last time you saw your favorite NFL star standing in a slumped posture with his head and shoulders rounded forward? Top athletes, generally have good posture partly because strong muscles from the ground up make it easier and more efficient to stand erect and to compete at a higher level. Nature has selectively eliminated couch potato posture from the ranks of professional athletes.

Second, muscle strength is needed as a shield to prevent trauma to other parts of the body. Strong muscles supply dynamic protection to joints by providing addition-al stability, while taking stress off static structures like ligaments and cartilage. A rod case is a simple analogy of a protective muscle. It is an exterior structure that guards fragile rods from trauma during transportation. Strong muscle on the outside protects more fragile joints on the inside.

Third, muscles complement each other's opposing forces producing a smooth, balanced motion of a joint. Dynamic balanced strength in all of the shoulder muscles is critical for healthy long-term use. If the deltoid muscle is too strong and the rota-tor cuff muscles are too weak, the imbalance leads to early wear and tear to the rota-tor cuff tendons. Balance is a universal good quality that is not only good for our shoulder function, but also for family relationships. Think of muscles as separate indi-viduals in the family. Each one has an important role in the family and needs a given amount of attention and worth or the whole system fails. We guarantee that spend-ing equal time and energy with all family members will also prolong your fishing time. Just as some crazed fishermen spend every waking moment on the water and eventually lose their wife and children, a strong deltoid by itself looks good from the outside, bu, overpowers the rotator cuff muscles resulting in early collapse of the "shoulder family".

Fourth, strong muscles produce about 85 percent of the body's total heat output. A hot body burns more calories at rest making it easier to keep body fat to a mini-mum so you can keep looking good in those tight fitting waders!

Strength can be improved in muscle more efficiently by controlling three impor-tant parameters of exercise including frequency, intensity, and duration. Strength training exercise should be performed 3-4 days per week minimum. The intensity of the exercise should be increased gradually by adding more weight or tension as tol-erated so the muscle becomes fatigued by the end of the last set. Increasing the inten-sity of an exercise is one of the best ways to improve pure strength in a muscle. Duration may be increased by adding more repetitions per set (increase from 3 sets of 10 reps, to 3 sets of 15 reps), or more sets per session (4 sets of 10 reps). Increasing the duration is an effective way to add endurance to any muscle.

Bodyblade®

The fly-fishing cast requires repetitive movement of the arm through a fairly small range of motion, using accurate control with good strength and excellent endurance. The Bodyblade® is a unique patented exercise device that was invented by Bruce Hymanson to help rehabilitate his physical therapy patients and was released on the market in 1991. It was designed to strengthen the core muscles that support the cervical and lumbar spine, in addition to the shoulder muscle groups. We feel it is the best exercise device on the market for simulating the specific core and extremity demands of the fly-casting motion. We have included several exercises at the end of each treatment chapter which will enhance your rehab and improve your fishing performance.

The Bodyblade® is a patented flexible foil with small weights at each end and a soft hand grip in the middle of the shaft. With just a little bit of encouragement, the ends are designed to "oscillate" back and forth at a steady rate of 270 times per minute. Muscles and joints work quickly through a small range of motion against the force of inertia. While the rate of oscillation stays the same, the intensity of the workout can be increased by increasing the amplitude of the blade motion.

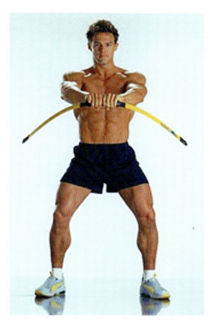

Bodyblade® in motion.

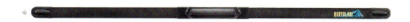

Full-length view of the Bodyblade®.

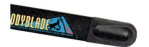

Tip weight.

It is a reactive device that only responds to the amount of force that you put into it. This feature makes it safe to use early in rehab as you can keep the level of resistance light at first to avoid pain production. As you gain strength, more force can be applied by increasing the size of motion to further challenge muscle strength and control. In addition, there are several different-sized blades which make it easy to closely match different body sizes and needs.

Bodyblade® Selection chart

Male: Excellent to Good Range					
Body Wt.	Pro	Classic	CXT	Cardio	Lite
150+ lbs.	**	*			
125-150 lbs.	**	*			
Child-125 lbs.	*	**	*		

Male: Fair to Sedentary					
Body Wt.	Pro	Classic	CXT	Cardio	Lite
150+ lbs.	*	**	*		
125-150 lbs.	*	**	*		
Child-125 lbs.		*	**		

Female: Excellent to Good Range					
Body Wt.	Pro	Classic	CXT	Cardio	Lite
150+ lbs.	**	*			
100-150 lbs.	*	*			
Child-100 lbs.			**	*	

Female: Fair to Sedentary					
Body Wt.	Pro	Classic	CXT	Cardio	Lite
150+ lbs.	*	**	*		
100-150 lbs.	*	**	*		
Child-100 lbs.			*	**	*

Strongly Recommended: **

Recommended: *

One of the first things you will notice while exercising with the Bodyblade® is that it not only works the targeted muscle group of that specific exercise, but also requires contraction of all other muscles throughout the entire body for stabilization. This means that there is a crossover benefit from one specific exercise to other muscle groups. For example, when performing the shoulder jab exercise, you are also strengthening muscles in the forearm, wrist, trunk, and legs. We will make reference to specific exercises in other chapters that may benefit your current problem.

Add one or two new exercises at a time to allow your muscles to adapt slowly. Exercise 3-5 times a week minimum. Try to start with 15 seconds of continuous motion during each exercise and gradually progress to 60 seconds as tolerated. Rest at least 30 seconds between each exercise. Intensity can be increased over time by moving the blade through a larger amplitude or by elevating it further away from your body. A detailed video is included with each purchase and covers this information in more depth.

We have made an arrangement with the Bodyblade ® Company to provide a 10% discount to purchasers of this book. Just include this code **(ESHIS0405080)** in the ordering process at Bodyblade.com or when phoning at 1-800-772-5233 to receive the discount on any of their products. We think you will find it an exceptional tool for improving your fishing performance!

Combining Treatment Methods and Progressing Rehab

Now that you have the tools, when and how do you use them? This is the most difficult aspect of self-treatment, but it has a huge impact on the speed of healing and your end results. Rehabilitating a torn hamstring muscle by pumping out hamstring curls at the gym with fifty pounds of weight guarantees failure and prolongs recovery. Ligament injuries, on the other hand, can often handle early strengthening of the surrounding muscles through a limited range of motion. Combining the correct treatment techniques at the appropriate time makes a world of difference.

Start to evaluate each new ache or pain as if you were a doctor in the emergency room. They are trained to triage injuries as they come through the door and will prioritize them by severity or need for further diagnostic tests. For instance, any ache or pain which is the result of a sudden traumatic injury should direct you immediately to your doctor for further testing and diagnostics.

> *For instance, any ache or pain which is the result of a sudden traumatic injury, should direct you immediately to your doctor for further testing and diagnostics.*

Many traumatic injuries involve enough force to completely tear internal joint structures which are not visible on the outside, and will not heal with rest and exercise alone. These injuries will often require further diagnostic tests, like x-rays or an MRI (Magnet Resonance Imaging), to see inside the joint and detect damage. Many of these traumatic injuries require immediate surgery, casting, or splinting for maximum healing to occur. You may jeopardize your chances for a complete recovery if you ignore getting a complete evaluation and or appropriate treatment first.

If your pain came on slowly over a period of time while performing a repetitive activity, then you have most likely developed an overuse injury. These types of injuries usually do not involve a complete tear of a joint structure, so they can be treated more conservatively at first with home-based treatment programs such as those outlined in this book. Progress should be seen in the first month with application of these conservative treatments. If you are not making progress during the first month of treatment, then it is time to see your doctor or therapist for more advice. Some aches and pains that come on slowly are related to a more serious internal illness which can refer pain to the limbs. These types of problems may be constant day and night, and are not made better or worse with change in joint position or movement. Many of these problems will have other symptoms like nausea, fever, chills, or fatigue which can be indicators of a more serious condition.

One huge misconception instilled by people in sports medicine and therapists alike is "no pain, no gain". Never has one saying harmed so many, because it is often applied to the wrong injury or at the wrong time. Now granted, I've inflicted my fair share of pain to patients as a therapist, but applying this mentality to *every* ache and pain that comes along is doomed to failure. When used inappropriately, "if it hurts, don't do it", is equally harmful. Each concept maximizes healing when applied correctly. Learning what not to do is an important concept in rehabilitation. These concepts will also be discussed in greater detail in later chapters.

It is important to *stretch* only to the point of pain, and not beyond. On the other hand, most tight joints will not improve unless stretch is taken to that point of pain and held there. This is an appropriate application of the concept, *"no pain no gain"*. If sharp pain occurs with any *strengthening* exercise, reduce the intensity, modify the range of motion, or drop the exercise until it can be performed without sharp

> *It is normal to have some increase in the level of soreness and ache while stretching or strengthening an injured part, but this elevated pain level should gradually taper off to a pre-exercise level in less than one hour.*

pain. This is an appropriate application of the concept, "if it hurts, then don't do it".

Learning to listen to your body during all stages of recovery prevents overdoing or underdoing exercise. It is normal to have some increase in the level of soreness and ache while stretching or strengthening an injured part, but this elevated pain level should gradually taper off to a pre-exercise level in less than one hour.

If it remains at an elevated level, then the next exercise session needs to be shorter, less intense, or less frequent. This will allow time for tendons, ligaments, and muscles to adapt to lighter loads. You can then try to increase the loads again after a week or two of exercising at these lighter levels. Less is more!

4
CHAPTER

Shoulder Impingement Syndrome

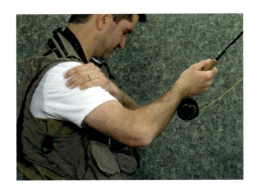

Introduction

As my (Dr. Berend's) old professor liked to say, "the shoulder is like an onion". It has layers and layers, they are all interconnected, they function together, but each layer has its own complexity, its own problems. We would have to agree. The shoulder represents, perhaps, one of the most complex joints in the body. With its complexity comes a myriad of possible aliments. With each ailment, multitudes of possible solutions exist. It has but one function: to position the hand in space. Yet, it has the greatest and most complex range of motions of any joint in the body. To substantiate this bold statement, the shoulder has four separate joints, four supporting layers of tissues, and seventeen muscles that attach to the shoulder blade. Each acts in concert to move the arm in ways and directions not obtainable by other joints in the body. It is easy to imagine that with all these parts and motions, the shoulder can have many, many problems. While oversimplified, the common reasons for shoulder problems can be boiled down to the Four Horsemen of shoulder ailments: bursitis, impingement, instability, and arthritis. These can be intermingled with or independent of each other. See, very complex! Add to that the complexity of the fly-cast, and we have an almost impenetrable combination of problems to discuss.

Symptoms

This is a list of some common symptoms experienced with this impingement syndrome. You may have some or all of these symptoms depending on the severity of your condition.

- Constant dull ache in the front or side of shoulder.
- Ache radiates from the upper arm to the elbow.
- Pain in the shoulder when lifting arm overhead or out to the side, especially in mid range.
- Pain worsens with start of activity and may decrease with use.
- Pain worsens at rest after prolonged use of the arm.
- Pain when reaching arm across chest.
- Pain when reaching arm back to put hand in coat sleeve.
- Pain reaching behind back to scratch an itch or place wallet in back pocket.
- Tip of shoulder tender to touch.

Description

Impingement syndrome is defined as inflammation of the shoulder's rotator cuff, bicep's tendon, or bursa. This may be due to poor shoulder mechanics, overuse, poor posture, weakness, or tightness. Your average run-of-the-mill impingement syndrome usually involves several of these factors.

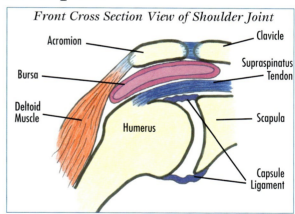

Front Cross Section View of Shoulder Joint

Acromion — Clavicle — Supraspinatus Tendon — Bursa — Deltoid Muscle — Humerus — Scapula — Capsule Ligament

Contributing Factors

For the avid long-rodder, there exists unanswered questions and mysteries in fly-fishing that may never be fully understood: entomology, feeding behaviors, and spawning activity. Perhaps the most vexing is why fish bite this day and not that day, but these intricacies of our sport draw many of us to the stream, day in and day out. It is these mysteries that some believe are the roots of fly-fishing itself, those unanswered questions that keep us interested in the fly, the fish, and the fishery. The same can be said of orthopedics. Some questions and problems have straightforward answers: bone broke: fix bone. Yet there remain others for which we, as clinicians, do not have all the answers. The shoulder is one of those conundrums. When you look at the mechanics and kinematics (the description of joint motion using mechanics to help understand forces developed across a joint) of the fly-cast, you can quickly see that the shoulder does most of the work. And it shows! In my (Dr. Berend's) study of the orthopedic problems of people who fly-fish, twenty-four percent of people reported shoulder problems related to fly-fishing. Thus, a quarter of those who fish suffer from one or more of their *onion layers* gone bad.

> ## *Thus, a quarter of those who fish suffer from one or more of the onion layers gone bad.*

A large study of musculoskeletal disorders in the work place, found that the most common risks for shoulder problems were from highly repetitive rhythm, significant use of force, awkward postures (overhead work), and specific actions of shoulder flexion and abduction (use of arm up front or out to the side). Sound familiar? That pretty much describes the typical day on the trout stream or a typical day hunting for bonefish. The authors of that study also concluded that increased muscle contraction leads to fatigue and possibly increased problems. So, it is not surprising that my study also showed that thirty-one percent of people who saltwater fly-fish (longer casts, heavier tackle) had shoulder pain, while twenty-three percent of those who trout fish had shoulder pain.

If there were a contest to design a sport that would most quickly lead to impingement syndrome injury to the shoulder, fly-fishing would certainly place in the top ten. The optimum strategy to irritate the shoulder involves several important components of motion and in the right amounts. First, you would want to position the upper arm so that it was out away from the side. This position narrows the space in the shoulder joint so there is little room for the tendons, causing the greatest amount of impingement or pinching of those tendons. Second, you would want to impart a rotational motion to that upper arm so as to grind the impinged tendons to a pulp. Third, you would want to perform that motion repeatedly over several hours so as to impart the most micro trauma possible to the tendon fibers, resulting in frayed tendons that could not possibly recover in one day.

These three conditions have been fully met with fly-fishing. Throw in some bad casting habits, extremely windy conditions, weak and deconditioned muscles, and an eight-weight rod, and you have a disaster waiting to happen. It's amazing that so many people participate in the sport for so many years prior to developing shoulder pain.

Primary Impingement: The Tight Bearing

Think of the shoulder as a wheel bearing joint. If you have ever over-tightened a wheel bearing on your car, you know that extra tension leads to early wear of the bearing and eventual failure.

Most bearings have a specific tightness or torque setting with which they operate most efficiently. On the other hand, too loose, and the bearing has extra slop with the same end results.

> *Think of the shoulder as a wheel-bearing joint. If you have ever over-tightend a wheel bearing on your car, you know that extra tension leads to early wear of the bearing and eventual failure.*

People cursed with very tight ligaments and deep joints are more susceptible, because the ball does not have enough room available in the socket during overhead reach—the *too tight* bearing scenario. In addition, a large overhanging or downwardly hooked Acromion, a bony part of the scapula which forms the top of the shoulder socket, predisposes the genetically unlucky to the same problem. These types of impingement are classified as *primary impingement syndrome.* This tightness may be due to a long winter in front of the TV where the hand is never lifted above the mouth. It may be the result of aging in which there is a loss of *Elastin,* a springy connective tissue in tendons and ligaments, and subsequent, gradual shortening of those soft ligaments. In this case, aging refers to anyone over twenty five—the approximate age when Elastin loss begins.

Secondary Impingement: The Loose Bearing

Secondary impingement syndrome occurs in those blessed with loose ligaments and flexible joints, but weak muscles. In this case, tendons are still impinged in the same location, but for a different

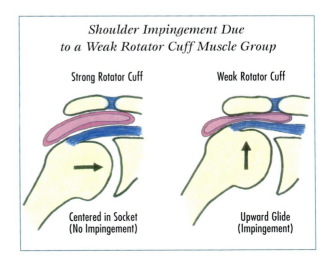

Shoulder Impingement Due to a Weak Rotator Cuff Muscle Group

Strong Rotator Cuff

Weak Rotator Cuff

Centered in Socket (No Impingement)

Upward Glide (Impingement)

mechanical reason—the too-loose bearing scenario. The rotator cuff and shoulder blade muscles are too weak to stabilize the ball in the center of the socket, so the ball rides up in the socket during overhead reach and impinges the tendons.

An imbalance can exist for two reasons: 1. The cuff muscles are allowed to atrophy, or weaken, with inactivity. 2. The large deltoid or biceps muscles are strengthened and the smaller cuff muscles are ignored during strength training. Over development of the large muscles often occurs in body-builders and weight-lifters who focus on major muscle group strengthening and forget about the smaller, non-visible rotator cuff muscles. When the deltoid is stronger and overpowers the cuff, it tends to win the tug of war during arm elevation, causing the ball to be jammed instantly upward into the Acromion bone before the weaker cuff muscles have the chance to stabilize the ball in the center of the socket. The stronger deltoid will win over the short haul, but eventually will surrender to the pain that emanates from its neighbors, the rotator cuff tendons that reside immediately downstairs. The body rewards balanced teamwork and penalizes individual standouts. Specific strengthening exercises need to be performed to the rotator cuff muscles to avoid this imbalance when strength training.

When cuff tendons are repeatedly irritated by grinding between the ball and socket bones, i.e. the humeral head and the Acromion process, they become painful, red, swollen, and frayed. If inflammation continues a long time, fibrosis will begin to form in the tendon and lay down new scar tissue and extra collagen effectively thickening it. These thick tendons can then take up more room in an already tight space and further the cycle of impingement.

Overtraining

Balance is rewarded when you slowly increase the rate of work a tendon performs. Tendonitis is frequently seen in runners' knees when they increase the number of miles run in preparation for a longer race. Tendons trained to handle running twenty miles per week will become inflamed and break down if the running is suddenly increases to forty miles a week. For this same reason, tendonitis can easily develop in the shoulder if sudden, increased demands are placed on it. A dramatic increase in the number of hours you fish per day, or the number of days you fish per week, will have the same impact.

A gradual increase in use of the shoulder in preparation for the first of the season allows the shoulder to adapt slowly to those demands, resulting in less chance of tendonitis. A good rule of thumb when increasing activity of any kind is to progress that activity by no more than ten percent per week.

> **A good rule of thumb when increasing activity of
> any kind is to progress that activity by
> no more than ten percent per week.**

This gives the body adequate time to adapt to changes and become stronger. Fishing for two hours the first day out and adding time slowly over several weeks can help prevent problems. Obviously this is nearly impossible to control if the first day out involves a spectacular caddis hatch lasting from 1 P.M. until 5 P.M. Training with the following exercises starting at least a month before a big trip or the start of the season can achieve the same results.

Scapula: A Stable Foundation

Further support can be obtained by adding strength to the foundation of the upper arm, which is the scapula. This *chicken wing*, or shoulder blade, provides a stable platform from which the upper limb operates. It contributes about one third of the available range seen in overhead motions. If the muscles that hold the scapula solidly against the trunk are weak, then the scapula is allowed to slump down and rotate forward in a protracted position. So, no big deal, right? Wrong! This forward position lets the ball ride forward in the socket where it receives less support by the mechanical shape of the socket and surrounding ligaments. Thus, it

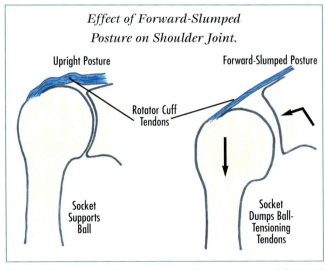

Effect of Forward-Slumped Posture on Shoulder Joint.

Upright Posture   Forward-Slumped Posture

Rotator Cuff Tendons

Socket Supports Ball

Socket Dumps Ball-Tensioning Tendons

allows the arm to hang entirely by the supporting tendons. This constant, additional load to the cuff muscles leads to early wear and tear.

A forward-rotated scapula essentially uses up some of the available range at the ball-and-socket so that the arm stops at an earlier point when attempting to reach overhead. This effect can be illustrated by standing bent forward at the waist at about a forty-five-degree angle, and then attempting to reach a top shelf. Overhead motion is diminished due to the forward angle of the scapula.

Hunched-Back Posture

While on this subject, we would be remiss if we did not mention that the scapula and upper back operate together. This means that if your upper back is hunched forward, looking like the Hunchback of Notre Dame, the scapula has also followed this plane of forward sloping, creating a forward shoulder blade position. All of these same problems can arise at the ball-and-socket of the shoulder joint when the upper back is leaning forward. Mom knew more about good fishing posture than we gave her credit for.

Traumatic Onset

Traumatic tendonitis is more difficult to prevent because it can occur with any forceful blow to the shoulder or fall on an outstretched arm. The fall jams the shoulder joint together, effectively bruising or tearing the tendon. After trauma to the body, soft tissues respond first by initiating the inflammation process, which starts to heal the injured area. Left unchecked and with further irritation, i.e. false casting all day, the inflammation process may spread beyond its initial confines and encroach on adjacent tissues.

Early treatment is critical in controlling inflammation and confining it to the original soft tissues that were traumatized. If you fall hard on your shoulder while descending a slippery bank, it is good preventative medicine to ice that bruised shoulder as soon possible. Taking two to four ibuprofen tablets right away, and then every six to eight hours the next day, can keep the inflammation in check until ice is available. Always remember to take ibuprofen with food, and stop taking it if gastro-intestinal discomfort develops. The adage "an ounce of prevention is worth a pound of cure" applies when dealing with fresh injuries. Treating injuries early on can greatly diminish the spread of inflammation to other tissues and therefore decrease their longevity and severity of an injury. Missing only one afternoon of fishing is easier treatment to swallow than missing an entire month of fishing.

Casting and Fishing Modifications

Move Closer

Fly-casting can provoke shoulder pain, so there should be something about the act of casting that you can modify to minimize the wear and tear on your shoulder. For starters, move closer to your target so that your cast is as short as possible. Forty five feet of line out requires substantially more load and range of motion from the shoulder than casting twenty feet. When stream fishing, this has the added benefit of catching more fish because of better targeting and less drag.

Start Slowly

Keep the frequency and duration of your fishing to a lower level at the beginning of the season to allow time for your shoulder to adapt slowly to these new loads. If you're already in pain, keep a tight reign on your fishing time and frequency so that you prevent progression of your overuse injury to a severe level. The less time you fish injured, the more time you have for treatment.

Keep it Hot

A warm shoulder will function better than a cold shoulder. Unfortunately, there are no good shoulder supports that you can wear to facilitate protection of your shoulder while fishing. Your best bet will be to keep your shoulder well insulated with a jacket that retains body heat and blocks the wind. Additionally, before you head out to the river, you should pre-heat shoulder muscles by performing the strengthening exercises listed at the end of this chapter. There is no better way to warm-up a muscle than by forcing it to burn some calories during strengthening exercises.

Elbow Down and Chest Out

Keeping the elbow lower down towards your side is another handy practice. This arm position effectively provides more room for the rotator cuff tendons under the Acromion. More room means less impingement with casting. Long casts require a higher elbow, while shorter casts can be made with a lower elbow.

> ### Resist the urge to stoop forward at the waist while hunting rising trout.

Stand tall with your chest out and shoulder blades pulled backward slightly, and the shoulder joint will function better with less impingement. Resist the urge to stoop forward at the waist while hunting rising trout.

I think we naturally assume this hunter/predator posture when casting to visible or rising fish because we believe they can see us more easily as well. While this may be true in some down-and-across presentations, most fish are spooked by our rod, line, or presentation, rather than by our body profile.

Use the Whole Body

Stand with one foot forward and one foot back while keeping both knees slightly bent to increase the amount of power generated from your legs and trunk, rather than from the shoulder alone. If you are a right-handed caster, then you should place the left foot out in front. Placing the body in this position promotes the use of trunk and leg muscles allowing them to contribute more to the casting power. Additionally, this position allows the shoulder to generate power from the middle of its range of motion where impingement is the least prevalent. To demonstrate this to yourself, start casting in your normal standing position. Then cast while kneeling on the right knee with the left foot on the ground, and finally from kneeling on both knees. This progression gradually eliminates the lower body from the cast, thereby increasing the power and range required from the shoulder. In this same vein, you should cast from a standing position while fishing from a drift boat. Seated casting may be more relaxing, but removes power from the legs and trunk forcing the shoulder to work harder.

Grab a Lighter Rod

Use the lightest rod that will do the job in the conditions you're fishing. As you know, rod and line weight add significantly to arm loading while casting and can have a big impact on shoulder health. Fishing on a windy day is one of the only situations where a slightly heavier rod may be easier on the shoulder, because you can punch the line through the wind more easily with a heavier line and stiffer rod. The extra weight of the rod and line is over-shadowed by the increased power that this rod can generate. Along these same lines, fishing a weight-forward line will load a rod more easily than a double taper line, allowing easier casting in the wind. I (Steve) frequently find myself changing up from a three-weight to a five-weight rod when the wind kicks up while out on the Madison River.

A few simple changes in technique can radically decrease loads to the shoulder. After applying these principals, beware of the new temptation to fish a longer day.

Treatment

We are not attempting to diagnose or treat any specific ailment, and we encourage you to seek medical attention for any significant complaint you may have that does not respond to self-help care. In addition, if your pain is the result of a fall or lifting injury, you should have your shoulder evaluated first by an orthopedist or physical therapist.

So where do you start? Remembering the basics of therapy can be a big help when dealing with any problem, especially impingement syndrome. If it's inflamed, then ice and rest it. If it's tight, then stretch it. If it's weak, then strengthen it. If it's healing, then friction massage it. These principals can all be applied to the treatment of a painful shoulder.

Manual therapy treatment provided by a physical therapist is a means to regain motion in an excessively tight shoulder. This treatment may include joint mobilization and passive stretching to restore lost motion when you are unable to make sufficient progress on your own. Many shoulder problems may have other structural problems which will require surgery to fully maximize recovery. Consult with a physical therapist or shoulder surgeon if your progress stalls while performing this program.

1. **Rest:** Cut back any activity that causes pain by at least fifty percent. Use the extra time to perform exercise and treatment options listed below. Once the pain is absent and you're tolerating all of the exercises listed below, gradually add in fishing time by no more than ten percent per week.

2. **Anti-inflammatory Medications:** Take Ibuprofen or Naproxen Sodium (Aleve) at the dose prescribed on the bottle for the first few days after an acute injury, or for up to fourteen days with a chronic injury. Take these medications day and night to keep them in your system to maximize the reduction of pain and inflammation. Take with food and discontinue use if stomach or gastrointestinal discomfort develops.

3. **Friction Massage:** Rub the painful areas of the shoulder for five minutes, one to two times a day. (See the description of transverse friction massage on page 19 for details). Make sure to move the skin back and forth, rather than sliding the fingertips over the skin. Gradually increase the downward pressure as the soreness decreases.

4. **Ice Massage:** Move the ice cup over the painful top of the shoulder for eight to ten minutes, one to two times a day. (See description of ice massage on page 18 for details). Always use ice after you exercise, or at the very end of the day. An alternative is to apply an ice pack for twenty minutes.

5. **Stretching:** Perform each exercise below 5-10 times, hold each stretch for a minimum of 30 seconds, and perform all exercises 2-3 times a day. Stretch to the point of pain and not through it. A stretch of long duration and low intensity is more effective in regaining lost motion than is an intense, short stretch.

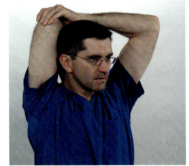

Arm Behind Head: Reach arm overhead, bend elbow and try to touch upper back with your hand. Place the hand of the uninjured arm on the injured elbow and pull arm behind head.

Arm Across Chest: Lift arm straight up in front of chest to shoulder level, use good hand to grab injured elbow, and pull upper arm across

Arm behind head stretch.

chest, moving elbow towards opposite shoulder. Move elbow up or down slightly to find the position of best stretch and least pain.

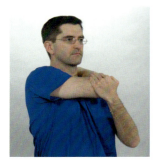

Overhead Stretch: Stand in open doorway and reach up the doorjamb as far as your shoulder allows. Increase stretch by leaning forward into the doorjamb. Rotate the hand in or out to find the most pain free position of stretch.

Arm across chest stretch.

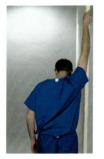

Overhead stretch.

Standing External Rotation Stretch: Stand in an open door with arm at side and elbow bent to ninety degrees. Place palm on doorjamb, rotate upper body away from that side, allowing your arm to twist outward. If this produces sharp shoulder pain, then back off on the intensity of stretch, or drop it and try the door pectoral stretch described below.

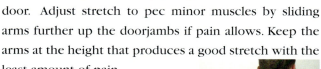

Standing Door Pectoral Stretch: Stand in open doorway, reach up and out, placing forearms on doorjambs. Step one foot through the door, keep stomach muscles tight, and lean through door. Adjust stretch to pec minor muscles by sliding arms further up the doorjambs if pain allows. Keep the arms at the height that produces a good stretch with the least amount of pain.

External rotation shoulder stretch.

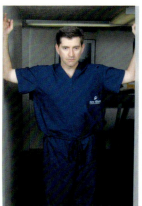

Door pec stretch.

Standing Towel Internal Rotation Stretch: Stand with towel in good hand. Drape towel over shoulder and reach injured arm up behind back and grab towel. Use towel to pull injured arm up behind back. Stop at point of pain or stretch.

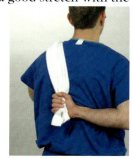

Towel internal rotation stretch.

6. Strengthening Exercises: Specific exercises can help you build up the layers of the onion, and keep the Four Horsemen from ruining your next outing. As with any exercise program, you should do these after adequate warm-up. Use high numbers of repetitions and low weight to tone and condition the target muscles. You can do them everyday if you use light weights and do not have a progressive increase in pain. Rotator cuff muscles primarily function as stabilizers, which require prolonged, constant contraction and good endurance. Remember that we are training for fly-fishing, not the Olympics!

> *Rotator cuff muscles primarily function as stabilizers, which require prolonged, constant contraction and good endurance.*

Perform exercises slowly and controlled in both directions for maximum strength gains and safety. Start with 3x15 reps (3 sets of 15 repetitions) for each exercise. Take a 30-second break between each set to allow the muscles to restore their oxygen levels.

Once an exercise becomes well tolerated with little fatigue, increase to 4x20 reps, rather than adding more resistance. Remember that these are primarily endurance muscles. Do not overload resistance in any exercise to the point where you are unable to complete the last set.

Rubber Band Exercises: The remaining strengthening exercises can be performed using a six-foot piece of rubber band or. Theraband®, a registered trademark of the Theraband Company, is a rubber band material available in many different thicknesses that allow for progressive increases in resistance. This material is usually stocked by physical therapists. We recommend using a six-foot length of the blue colored, medium-strength band because it has the right amount of resistance for shoulder work. Some of these exercises can also be performed using dumbbells or adjustable weight cuffs. They will be described below as an option for some exercises. Each of the following exercises should be performed slowly both in the shortening and lengthening motions. If one part of the range of motion is painful, avoid working in that range, or concentrate on a smaller range that is comfortable. Avoid an exercise if you are unable to find a comfortable range to work in. Try to add it in later as pain decreases. Once you are able to perform 4x20 reps with good control, add tension by using a shorter section of band, or by pre-tensioning the band.

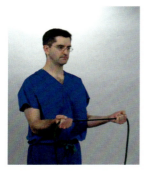

External rotation.

External Rotation: Grab the band with both hands. With elbows bent to ninety degrees and against your sides, pull both arms out slowly. The shoulder may be more comfortable with a small towel roll placed under armpit. A similar exercise can be performed with a dumbbell. Lie down with the non-injured side against the floor, injured elbow bent and resting on the top side of the rib cage. Then lift the hand upwards towards the ceiling. Start off with 3x15 reps, and then increase to 4x20 reps as tolerated.

Internal Rotation: Tie a small loop in one end of the band and place it around a doorknob. Keeping elbow bent to ninety degrees, grab the end and pull it across your chest. A small towel roll under the armpit may help reduce pain.

Start off with 3x15 reps, and then increase to 4x20 reps as tolerated.

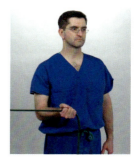

Internal rotation.

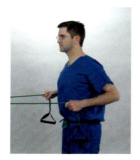

Rowing.

Rowing: Loop the center of band around a doorknob with the door open. Grab one end with each hand while sitting in a chair. Pull hands back to sides/ribs, and try to pinch shoulder blades together. Keep upper back straight and stationary. Start off with 3x15 reps, and then increase to 4x20 reps as tolerated.

Standing Abduction: Stand on one end of the band with other foot, and grab the end of the band with injured hand. Lift arm out from side, keeping palm in position of maximum comfort. Do not lift any higher than shoulder level. Rotate the arm in or out to find a comfortable position. You may use a dumbbell or cuff weight in the same manner.
Perform 3x15 reps.

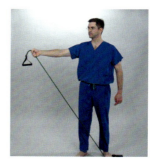

Standing abduction.

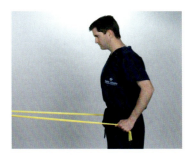

Standing extension.

standing Extension: Loop the center of the band around a doorknob. Grab the other ends with your hands. Lift your arms backwards, keeping your thumb pointed out, pull back to hip level. Start off with 3x15 reps, and then increase to 4x20 reps as tolerated.

Forward-Bent Kneeling Row: Lean forward over a couch or chair supporting your weight with your good arm and knee. Stand on one end of the band, and grab the other end with your injured hand. Pull your hand up to side of ribs while bending elbow. Use dumbbell or cuff weight in the same manner. Start off with 3x15 reps, and then increase to 4x20 reps as tolerated.

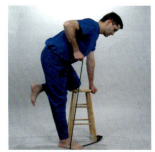

Forward-bent kneeling row.

Advanced Strengthening Exercises

Once the previous exercises become comfortable, add the following to your program.

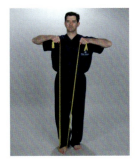

Upright row.

Upright Row: Stand with feet together on the center of the band, and grab the band in each hand. Lift hands and elbows to shoulder level while bending elbows. Use dumbbell or cuff weight in the same manner. Start off with 3x15 reps, and then increase to 4x20 reps as tolerated.

Front Lifts: Stand with thumbs pointing forward. Lift arms up in front of body to overhead position, keeping elbows straight. Lift as high as pain allows, i.e. stay below level that may cause pain. Use dumbbell or cuff weight in the same manner. Start off with 3x15 reps, and then increase to 4x20 reps as tolerated.

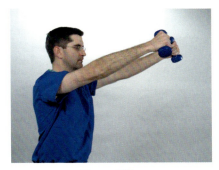

Front lifts.

Bodyblade® Exercises

General instructions: Start with continuous motion for 15 seconds and gradually add time towards a goal of 60 seconds. Add a second set to each exercise once you are able to complete all of the listed exercises with good control and no pain. The second set should be progressed from 15 seconds to a goal of 60 seconds in the same gradual manner. Rest at least 15-20 seconds between each exercise. Increase resistance on each exercise as tolerated by moving the blade with more force, producing an increased flex in the blade. Refer to page 28 for Bodyblade ordering information.

Chest Press:

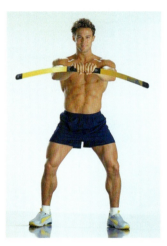

Stand with your feet at least shoulder width apart and knees slightly bent for good stability. Grab the handle with both hands palms facing down and looking at the flat edge of the blade. Move the blade forward and backward with a push/pull motion to produce a resistance that is challenging in each of the following positions:

A. Arms low with hands at around waist level. (Goal 2x60 seconds)

B. Arms high with hands at shoulder level as shown in picture. (Goal 2x60 seconds)

Chest Press High.

Jab:

Stand with your feet at least shoulder width apart and knees slightly bent for good stability. Grab the handle with one hand so that the flat edge of the blade is pointing towards you.

Move the blade in a jabbing motion while in each of the following positions:

A. Arm down with hand by side. (Goal 2x60 seconds)

B. Arm in front of body at 90°. (Goal 2x60 seconds)

C. Arm out to side at 90° (Goal 2x60 seconds)

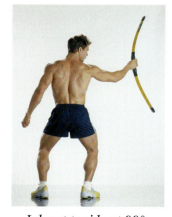

Jab out to side at 90°.

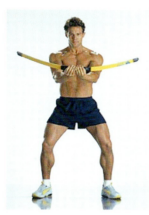

Bicep tricep curl.

Bicep Tricep Curl:

Stand with your feet at least shoulder width apart and knees slightly bent for good stability. Grab the handle with two hands, palms facing up and the flat edge of the blade facing towards you. Bend both elbows to about 30°. Drive the blade in and out with a push/pull motion. Goal 2x60 seconds.

Casting Simulation:

Add this exercise only after all of the exercises mentioned previously are well tolerated. Stand with one foot forward and one foot back with knees bent in a casting stance. Grab the handle with one hand so that the thin edge of the blade is pointing towards you. Lift your arm out to the side keeping the elbow bent and hand below shoulder level. Move the blade front to back to simulate the casting motion. Move your arm down and hand in front of your body if this position is painful. (Similar to rubber band external rotation position.) Goal 2x60 seconds.

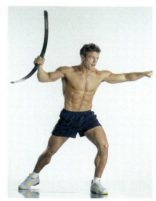

Casting simulation.

Shoulder Program	Date	Date	Date	Date	Date	Date	Date	Date	Date	Date
Arm Behind Head Stretch										
Arm Across Chest Stretch										
Overhead Stretch										
External Rotation Stretch										
Door Pec Stretch										
Towel Internal Rotation Stretch										
Band External Rotation										
Band Internal Rotation										
Band Rowing										
Band Abduction										
Band Extension										
Band Kneeling Row										
Band Upright Row										
Front Lifts										
Bodyblade Chest Press										
Bodyblade Jab										
Bodyblade Bicep/Tricep Curl										
Bodyblade Casting Simulation										

Make photocopies of this sheet to help you record your progress and stay disciplined with your exercise program.

Use this exercise flow sheet to record the date you performed each exercise. The top half of the sheet contains the name of each *stretching* exercise and a blank space to record the number of reps performed each day. Example: write in "5x" to indicate that 5 reps were performed.

The bottom half of the sheet contains each of the *strengthening* exercises with a blank space to record the number of reps and sets performed each day. Example: write "3x10" to indicate that 3 sets of 10 reps were performed. You can record the number of pounds used if dumbbells are used instead of a rubber band. Example: write "3/3x10" to indicate 3 pounds of weight used during 3 sets of 10 reps.

[1] Prevalence of Orthopaedic Maladies in People Who Flyfish: An Internet-Based Survey
Keith R Berend, MD: *Journal of the Southern Orthopedic Association* 10:221-229, 2001

5
CHAPTER

Tennis Elbow and Golfer's Elbow

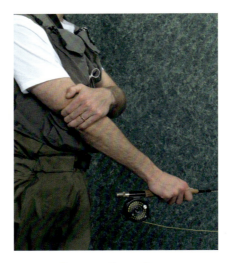

Introduction

The hinges on a door work well for what they do, allow the door to swing open and closed in one direction. The elbow, like a hinge, allows the lower arm (the forearm) to swing up and down and position the hand in space. However, unlike the simple, but effective, door hinge, the anatomy of the elbow is complex. With multiple muscles inserting and originating about the bony structures, the elbow is quite sensitive to overuse and repetitive motion. The most widely known and most diagnosed ailment is tennis elbow (lateral epicondylitis). Its bastard cousin, golfer's elbow (medial epicondylitis), is a similar condition that affects the hinge joint of the upper body. By virtue of the motion of the fly-cast and other activities we ask of our hinge during fishing, like rowing or carrying our gear, these conditions are frequently encountered by the angler. You don't have to play tennis or golf to suffer from these ailments. In fact, the majority of people afflicted by these conditions don't swing a club or racquet. It is likely that fishermen's elbow is a combination of tennis and golfer's elbow.

Tennis Elbow (Lateral Epicondylitis)

Symptoms

- Aching, burning, or sharp pain that lies over the outside of the elbow joint and may radiate to the wrist or back of the hand.
- The outer bony prominence of the elbow (lateral epicondyle) is tender to the touch.
- Grasping, making a fist, writing, lifting, or extending the wrist and fingers may increase pain.
- In severe forms, it may cause a constant ache at night, preventing sleep.

Description

Pain and inflammation of the *Extensor Carpi Radialis Brevis* tendon at its attachment to the outer bony prominence of the elbow, called the *Lateral Epicondyle*, gives us the name Lateral Epicondylitis. This tendon gives rise to a muscle that runs down the outside of the forearm to insert to the back side of the wrist and

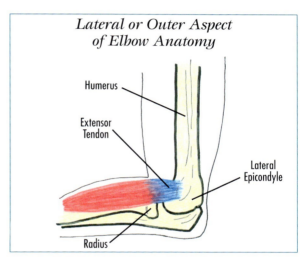

Lateral or Outer Aspect of Elbow Anatomy

Humerus

Extensor Tendon

Lateral Epicondyle

Radius

functions to bend the wrist backwards (extension). Overuse results in a breakdown of the tendon fibers at the elbow and leads to the body's attempt at healing the tendon by laying down more scar tissue in and around the tendon.

Golfer's Elbow (Medial Epicondylitis)

Symptoms

- Aching, burning, or sharp pain that lies over the inner aspect of the elbow joint and may radiate to the inner forearm.
- Tenderness to touch over the inner bony prominence of the elbow (*medial epicondyle*).
- Pain may increase with grasping, making a fist, flexing the wrist and fingers downward, twisting the wrist and forearm into a palm down position (pronation).
- In early and severe stages, this may cause a constant ache at night, preventing sleep.

Description

Pain and inflammation of the *Common Flexor Tendon* and *Pronator Teres Tendon* at its attachment to the inner bony prominence of the elbow (*Medial Epicondyle*), give it the name *Medial Epicondylitis*. These tendons give rise to muscles that run down the inner forearm and function to bend the wrist down (*flex-*

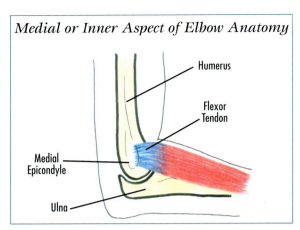

Medial or Inner Aspect of Elbow Anatomy

ion), or twist the forearm palm down (*pronation*). Overuse of these muscles results in a breakdown of the tendon collagen fibers where they attach to the inner elbow, resulting in the body's attempt to heal the tendon by laying down more scar tissue in and around the tendon.

General Contributing Factors for Both Areas

Many of us who have spent time beating the water with the long rod have suffered from elbow pain. While the majority of the time this is simply overdoing it, some fly-fishing enthusiasts suffer from what has been cleverly coined *fly-fishing elbow*. Fly-fishing elbow is obviously a spin-off of tennis elbow; a condition originally described 120 years ago. Regardless of definitions, fly-fishing elbow hurts, affects almost twenty percent of us from time to time, and can seriously interfere with our enjoyment of the sport. Now that we have a rough understanding of the cause of this persistent demon that plagues many of us, we will provide an overview of the common treatments that may help relieve the problem. Most importantly, a professional should evaluate any pain or medical condition from which someone suffers, and trained personnel should probably supervise initial treatment.

My perception is that fly-fishing elbow can be tennis elbow, golfer's elbow, or frequently a combination of both. "But why would I get fly-fishing elbow, I only fish for small fish with light rods?" you might question. Repetitive movements of the wrist and elbow pulling on the areas where these muscles attach to the elbow cause these conditions. Repetitive motions, such as casting the fly rod, flipping a casting rod, or hauling in a trophy, cause tiny tears in the tissues. These small tears don't necessarily cause pain while fishing—initially. However, continued overuse will prevent these areas from healing, and then scar tissue begins to develop. Scar tissue is painful, and prone to re-injury, more scarring, and more pain. This abnormal tissue eventually becomes very sore, and pain worsens when the muscles contract.

> *Scar tissue is painful, and prone to re-injury, more scarring, and more pain. This abnormal tissue eventually becomes very sore, and pain worsens when the muscles contract.*

The modern-day fishing enthusiast is at risk for these types of fishing maladies for several reasons. Age may be a factor; the average age of people who suffer from tennis elbow is forty to fifty years old, a common demographic seen hanging about the fly shop on Saturdays. However, anyone, of almost any age, can have tennis elbow. "Why me?" One of four factors or a combination of those factors brings on these conditions. First, an increase in the intensity of fly-fishing. This is the Keys flats guide who fishes a little bit a few hundred days a year, but during the steelhead season spends long hours for several days in a row doing the western Michigan chuck-and-duck. Other factors, such as rowing the boat during the busy summer terrestrial, season can be blamed as well, but the underlying factor is an increase in the intensity of the activity. Second is an increase in the frequency of fly-fishing. This is the case of the fly-fisherwoman who lives in Ohio and goes to New Jersey to fish a few times a year. She then retires and moves to New Jersey where she throws streamers for stripers six days in a row. The third factor is an increase in the duration of the activity. For example, a physician who lives in Montana and casts dry flies to spring creek trout a few evenings a month. He then takes a personal day to "find himself" on the trout stream and fishes all day. The final factor is poor conditioning. Without proper conditioning, the body's resistance to these insults is diminished and is at risk with any change in duration, frequency, or intensity.

My elbow hurts when I fish. Do I have epicondylitis? Other problems that mimic fly-fishing elbow include neck problems, like arthritis or a pinched nerve, arthritis of the elbow, gout in the elbow, or instability of the elbow. Many of these conditions can be exacerbated by fishing, so how is epicondylitis diagnosed? If the history is suggestive (the guide from the Keys, the women in New Jersey, or the doctor who found himself), then the physical exam is the next step. As described earlier, point tenderness over the lateral or medial epicondyle is pretty specific for these problems. Provocative tests, like grabbing the back of a dinner table chair with the palm down and lifting the chair, can cause an increase in the pain and is suggestive of tennis elbow (Lateral Epicondylitis). Increased pain with bending the fingers and wrist back towards the arm is suggestive of golfer's elbow (Medial Epicondylitis). Often grabbing and lifting motions, even light objects like a purse or plastic grocery bag can be painful. If there is swelling or tingling in the elbow or hand, then a source other than Lateral Epicondylitis should be sought. Numbness and tingling are occasionally associated with golfer's elbow, and these symptoms should prompt further examination. Catching, grinding, locking, and popping are not usually associated with tennis or golfer's elbow and should be evaluated by a doctor. If the history of onset is questionable, or if the physical findings are inconsistent with those we have described above, further work-up may be warranted.

Specific Causes of Tennis Elbow (Lateral Epicondylitis)

Fishing exposes the elbow to both bruises (traumatic tendonitis) and overuse tendonitis of the elbow. Overuse tendonitis is common to fly-fishermen. We just don't know when to stop fishing, especially when fish are rising to that blue-winged olive pattern. Personal experience has taught me that this is one circumstance that can sneak up on a guy in a hurry. Repeated false casting to air out a slightly damp dry fly can have disastrous consequences, making pain inevitable by the end of the day.

Next time you're out with your favorite fishing partner, take a close look at the joints that are moving the most, and you'll probably notice the elbow joint immediately. Much of the energy developed to cast a fly has its origin at the elbow joint as we're taught to move rod tip from the ten o'clock to the two o'clock position while keeping the wrist fairly still. The false cast requires a sudden deceleration of the rod at the ten o'clock position prior to the start of the back cast. This sudden stop requires excessive contraction in the muscles on the back and outside of the elbow which cross the wrist joint and produce this deceleration. Similarly, the sudden deceleration of the back cast at the two o'clock position requires a brief strong muscle contraction of the muscles that cross the inside and front of the wrist and elbow. These sudden stops also require the hand grasping muscles to squeeze the rod handle more firmly for just an instant. Visible motion at the elbow deceives most of us into thinking that it's this elbow movement that leads to soreness, when in fact, we need to look downstream at the wrist and hand to fully explain this particular overuse injury.

Wrist Back = Strong Grasp

For the hand to grasp any object firmly, the wrist needs to be positioned in an *extended* or backward bent position. This backward bent position is the primary job of the

Extensor Carpi Radialis Brevis muscle and its corresponding tendon. Improved grasp strength with the wrist in this position is due to the "tenodesis effect" and is easily illustrated by a little home anatomy science experiment.

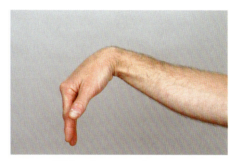

Wrist down weak grasp.

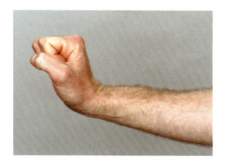

Wrist up strong grasp.

With your arm fully extended in front of you, and palm facing down, bend your wrist and hand downwards towards floor, then try and grasp one finger on your opposite hand with a strong grasp. While grasping the finger as hard as possible in this position, try to pull the finger free from the grasp. Pretty challenging to hang on to the finger with much gusto, huh? Now try the same thing, but instead of bending the wrist down into *flexion*, lift the wrist up into *extension* (towards ceiling). Voila! Your grasp strength has increased. You have proven that a backward bent wrist results in improved grip strength. The wrist extensor muscles that arise from the outside of the elbow need to contract strongly, pulling the wrist back in to extension, whenever the hand grasps a fly rod handle firmly. Overuse of this tendon is a direct result of a strong hand grasp to control the rod handle and to stabilize the wrist.

> *Overuse of this tendon is a direct result of a strong hand grasp to control the rod handle and to stabilize the wrist.*

Living Outside the Circle of Wagons

Physical location of the lateral epicondyle on the outer aspect of the body leads to the second, less frequent, cause of lateral epicondylitis. This location on the periphery of the body makes it more vulnerable to getting bumped, which can initiate the inflammation process. One of my (Steve's) past entrances into the Gallatin River came quickly as both feet slipped off a two-foot-high mud bank, launching me back and to one side. I landed hard on my butt and right elbow. Thank God a rock was there to stop my fall! That incident produced just enough trauma to get the inflammation process rolling. As I have stated before, inflammation can arise from a sharp bump to the elbow, traumatizing the tendon and starting the inflammation response. You are much less likely to bump the inside of your elbow (medial epicondyle) due to its location close to your body. This concept was quickly learned by the early settlers. It was safer living inside a circle of wagons than it was living outside the circle.

Specific Causes of Golfer's Elbow
(Medial Epicondylitis)

Tendonitis of the inner elbow is rarer than its lateral neighbor. As we discussed in the last section, much of the hand's grasp strength is developed by the extensor muscles on the back/outside of the forearm. Their function is to support the wrist in extension producing the tenodesis effect. Inward twisting of the forearm and wrist, as seen in a sidearm throw, is one of the movements that can cause golfer's elbow to flare up. This motion places a large strain on the medial elbow structures at the end of the cocking phase. Moving forward from this cocked position, the medial forearm muscles contract hard to partially twist the forearm from a palm-up to a palm-down position during forward acceleration. These muscles and tendons are under tremendous stress at the end of a forceful back cast, when the wrist and elbow must stop the backward motion of the arm and begin to propel the Woolly Bugger to its target.

Right-handed golfers often develop pain in the right elbow if they push the club down to the ball using the right hand and wrist, rather than pulling down with the left arm and trunk. Strong, fast wrist contraction to the ball overloads the medial tendons and eventually leads to pain, as well as a longer visit at the 19th hole to deaden the pain.

Similar forces are produced in fly-fishing when you increase the arm and trunk motion to cast line a greater distance. Lefty Kreh recognized the importance of allowing the shoulder and forearm to move back away from the body in order to increase casting distance. This larger movement of the arm increases the length of rod travel,

While effective at increasing distance, this casting style can allow more outward rotation of the forearm at the end of the back cast, placing greater stress to the medial side of the elbow.

and allows greater loading of the rod for more distance. While effective at increasing distance, this casting style requires more outward rotation of the forearm at the end of the back cast, placing greater stress to the medial side of the elbow. In addition, fishermen with tight shoulder joints that lack normal external rotation flexibility tend to compensate by using more forearm outward rotation motion on long casts which further overloads the inner elbow. This very effective casting stroke for longer casts requires balanced range of motion and strength from the entire arm to perform efficiently and without injury.

The forward phase of this cast starts with contraction of the muscles that twist the palm inward, while driving the forearm forward. Rotating the arm and shoulder out and back in this way increases torque, or twisting force, across the medial elbow which is controlled by the medial ligaments, muscles, and tendons. Since this casting motion is more prevalent in saltwater casters who require consistently longer casts with heavier equipment, you can see why they have almost twice the occurrence of elbow pain (30 percent) versus those who stalk their prey in warm water (12 percent), or cold water (16 percent) as was demonstrated by Dr. Berend's study.

Long-rodders can gain extra distance by performing a double haul while hunting tailing bonefish out on the flats. Pulling down with the line hand at just the right moment in the cast effectively bends the rod tip further, creating greater load in the rod which is then transferred to the line. Unfortunately, this increased rod load is also transferred downstream to the wrist and elbow. This "double haul" creates rod loading at both ends of the casting stroke and forces the muscles on both sides of the elbow to work overtime.

Picture a flag pole fixed in a dirt hole in the ground. If the tip of that pole is pulled back and the pole is bent, sooner or later the weak dirt foundation (the elbow) will

> *Extra strengthening and conditioning between seasons is the best method to combat these excessive loads.*

fail, and you'll be making an extra trip to Home Depot for a bag of concrete. Now, place that pole into concrete and bend it back. The same forces are transmitted down the pole to the base, but this time the foundation is strong enough to withstand the forces, and no failure occurs. Be the concrete! Extra strengthening and conditioning between seasons is the best method to combat these excessive loads.

Casting and Fishing Modifications

Many factors control how quickly overuse injury occurs in the elbow system. We have control over most of these factors, whether we choose to admit it or not. Frequency and duration of casting has a huge impact on how quickly tendons break down. An increase in either of these two variables increases the likelihood that you will develop tendonitis. Frequency involves both the number of casts we make in a given day, and the number of days we fish per week. The duration variable involves the number of hours in a row that we fish each outing.

Add Time Gradually

Adding time or frequency too quickly to an untrained arm has disastrous results. Runners who understand this training concept routinely restrict adding more than ten percent to their mileage in a given week. This rate of increase places new loads on the joints and tendons at a rate that allows time for them to adapt and avoid the production of overuse injuries. We often fail in this regard when we plan an extended fishing vacation that effectively doubles or triples the number of days per week that we cast. Begin to strengthen your arm months before a long fishing trip. Gradually increase weights and reps to prepare your arm for this heavier demand. This will build strength and endurance in arm muscles and tendons, preventing possible overuse injury. Early in the season you can avoid tendon breakdown by fishing three to four hours per day instead of eight, and/or rest a day after each day you fish.

Use the Whole Body

Overuse injury to the arm can be mitigated somewhat by changing casting technique. The greater the number of body parts we involve in the act of casting, the more we spread the loads to other joints. Standing at a forty-five-degree-angle to the casting target with one foot forward recruits more use out of the lower body and also encourages weight shift front to back as well as increased upper body rotation. Generating power from the trunk and legs in this fashion spreads the loads to other body parts making for a more fluid and powerful casting stroke.

Grab a Light Rod

There is a direct correlation of increased elbow loading as we grab a heavier rod/line weight. The longer and heavier the rod is, the greater the force developed in the arm during casting. Choose the lightest weight rod for the circumstances and you not only decrease the loads to the arm, but also increase the thrill of landing the fish. Wind is one occasion that requires a heavier rod and line to help punch the line appropriately with less effort.

Modern rods are a blessing and a curse. They allow us to keep more line in the air for longer casts, but may deceive us as we induce more damage to our musculoskeletal systems. Fishing stiff, high-modulus rods will often entice us to cast greater distances rather than move closer to the fish. We are deceived by a light rod in hand that is easy to lift and to cast repeatedly when compared to older, heavier rods. We have in essence exchanged rod weight for more stiffness and power which can be equally destructive if the rod is constantly being cast with a lot of line out.

Moving closer to our prey and making shorter casts reduces muscle/tendon loads at the hand, wrist, and forearm. Moving closer also allows a better chance to catch a rising fish, as each cast is more accurate, the dry fly is focused over the fish for a greater period of time and line drag is more easily eliminated.

Size Matters

Variables in the shape and size of the rod handle place different loads on elbow muscles and tendons. Smaller "superfine" cork handles taper down to the rod-blank diameter, allowing good "feel" on a smaller rod when casting to fish on a small stream at a short distance. One downside to this handle is less surface area of the palm and fingers in contact with cork, requiring greater hand grasp tension to control the rod. The other downside is that mechanical advantage of the tendons and muscles of the hand is decreased when grip size is reduced. This is fine at short distances, but casting at longer distances is impeded due to the increased loads required. A Full Wells cork handle places more surface area of the hand in contact with the cork, which lowers the loads per square inch required on the hand. Although this larger handle feels clunky at times, it does a better job of reducing stress to the elbow and wrist while casting at medium to longer distances.

There are small differences in optimum rod-grip diameter as determined by the length of one's fingers. Therapists use a grip strength dynamometer to evaluate hand injuries and document hand grip strength. This instrument has five test positions ranging from a small-sized grasp position to a large-sized grasp. A normal test result of all five positions creates a bell-shaped graph with the maximum hand strength developed at one of the middle test positions. This bell-shaped curve should be evident even in an injured or weakened hand, as it is influenced primarily by the ergonomic rules of muscle tendon length. Those with small hands are well advised to look for slightly smaller diameter cork grips to accommodate this smaller hand size. In the future, we may be able to walk into our local fly shop and have our hand casted or tested to determine the optimum shape and size of rod grip prior to building our new rod.

Stress reduction can be improved by modifying the cork grip in a rod that has an existing small grip design. Cork modification can be both expensive and a mess, depending on the rod design. A better alternative may be to modify your hand size.

This can be accomplished by wearing a glove or by wrapping the rod handle with tape. Fishermanshealth.com carries a high-quality fingerless glove that effectively increases grip size by adding a gel substance to the palm of the glove. Gel is located in the palm location and maximizes hand mechanical advantage while dampening shock transfer to the hand. A side benefit is less blister or callus formation in the palm.

Add a Rev-Limiter

Use of a counter-force brace on the forearm is yet another common way to reduce loads to the tendon. This works similarly to a rev-limiter on an engine in that it turns the muscle off before it contracts too forcefully, thus protecting the tendon. Placing one of these straps around the widest part of the forearm helps to restrict how hard the extensor tendon muscles contract during grasp activities. Three mistakes to avoid when applying the strap: 1. placing it on directly over the painful part of the elbow. This will cause more irritation to the tendon and it will not control the muscle contraction force. 2. putting it on too tightly. This severely limits the grasp and cuts off circulation to the forearm. The brace should be just tight enough to stay in position on the forearm so that when grasp occurs, muscular expansion creates a sense of pressure under the brace. 3. Wearing the brace every waking hour. Apply the brace only when you perform strong grasping activities. There is a danger of actually causing muscle weakness if the brace is worn all day, every day, because the muscle is not required to work at all. One additional caveat is that both good and not-so-good counter-force braces exist. The good ones have some type of bladder or padding that is applied over the target muscle groups to impact those groups more specifically than the ones not at risk. These pads or bladders can be air, foam, or special gels that lessen the vibration and stress on the muscle groups. These braces can be ordered online at Fishermenshealth.com or purchased locally. Bad braces are simply bands that tend to feel too tight and do not directly address the target muscle groups. These tend to feel more like a tourniquet than a support. Use of any brace should only be *part* of a complete treatment program. Stretching, strengthening, massage, and icing will round out a complete treatment program. They will actually change the underlying problem that is causing pain.

Overall, many changes can be made in technique and equipment to reduce stress to the elbow. We have the final say in many of these decisions and can implement changes quickly and easily. Often all that is required is that we step back, take a fresh look at how we fish, and make the appropriate changes.

Treatment

We are not attempting to diagnose or treat any specific ailment, and we encourage you to seek medical attention for any significant complaint that does not respond to self-help care.

An ounce of prevention is worth a pound of trout! Training the wrist and hand

An ounce of prevention is worth a pound of trout!

during the off-season helps to prevent these types of overuse injuries. A well-trained musculoskeletal system that has been maintained during the winter months can prevent many overuse injuries in the spring, as the muscles and their tendons have been kept at a higher level of fitness and strength. Avoiding falls on slippery rocks can reduce traumatic onset of tendonitis, but are more difficult to control or eliminate.

A huge range of pain and inflammation exists with lateral epicondylitis, and I (Steve) have seen the full spectrum in my practice over the years. The concrete-finishing business seems to produce some of the most painful patients because it requires a constant strong grasp, all-day motion, and working against a surface that gets progressively firmer. These guys come in with a constant throbbing ache in the elbow, forearm, wrist, and even in the upper arm. They haven't slept in a week and can barely hang on to their coffee cup by the time they see me. Needless to say, they are looking at a long, slow recovery and time off work to get things under control. The very severe cases will often require surgery or change in profession to alleviate the symptoms.

On the other end of the pain spectrum, I see the classic weekend gardener who works pruning and pulling weeds occasionally. They are living with a mild intermittent discomfort in the elbow which is only present while gardening. These people are pain-free soon after they stop gardening, and they can still perform ninety-five percent of their other tasks without pain. Certainly, these folks have not caused as much damage and will recover more quickly with less treatment than will the concrete finishers.

All of the self-care exercises described below should be applied to the treatment of either golfer's elbow or tennis elbow. It is important to stretch and strengthen both sides of an injured joint so forces are balanced across the joint.

The longer you have had the problem, the longer it will take to get rid of it. In other words, the sooner you catch and start to treat this problem, the sooner it will go away. Some severe cases may not respond entirely too conservative treatment and may need more involved treatment including ultrasound, manual therapy, injections,

> ## *The longer you have had the problem, the longer it will take to get rid of it.*

or as a last resort, surgery. Contact a local physical therapist or orthopedic surgeon if your progress stalls while using these suggestions.

1. **Protection:** As mentioned earlier, use of a counter-force brace on the forearm is a common way to reduce loads to the tendon.

   Placing one of these straps around the widest part of the forearm helps to restrict how hard the extensor tendon muscles contract during grasp activities. The brace should be just tight enough to stay in position

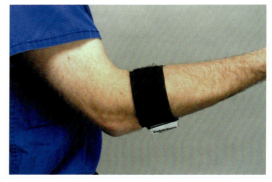

Elbow counterforce brace.

   on the forearm so that when grasp occurs, muscular expansion creates a sense of pressure under the brace. Apply the brace only during the period of time that strong grasping activities will be performed.

2. **Rest:** No matter where you fall along this spectrum, relative rest and protection are the first order of business. Giving the tendon a break from at least fifty percent of the amount of workload it has been performing is necessary to allow rebuilding of the injured fibers. The concrete finisher needs a larger dose of rest from his work and should stay away from his work continuously for a week or two to allow healing. The weekend gardener may get away with weeding only one day on the weekend rather than two. In any event, rebalancing your "treatment scale" is necessary for healing. Decrease the speed of breakdown on one side of the scale to allow treatment techniques on the opposite side of the scale to work their magic.

3. **Friction Massage:** Friction massage should be one of the early treatment techniques employed to begin stimulating increased blood flow and improve collagen qualities in the tendon. Obviously, the concrete finisher has a much higher level of tenderness and inflammation in his tendon and needs to start with lighter pressure and a shorter duration of massage than does the gardnerer. Using several fingertips over the tender areas, move the skin back and forth across the tendon

quickly in a direction that is perpendicular to the length of the tendon/muscle. As tenderness improves, gradually push deeper into the tendon, and lengthen the time that you massage towards a goal of 15 minutes. Perform friction massage 2-3 times per day as tolerated.

4. **Ice and Anti-inflammatory Medications:** Reducing inflammation in the extensor tendon can be accomplished using ice and anti-inflammatory medications frequently and consistently. Ice massage should be applied to the painful area of the elbow two to three times per day for about eight to ten minutes each session. Feel the burn! Ibuprofen or Aleve taken at the maximum dosage listed on the bottle for ten to fourteen days can make significant reductions in inflammation levels. Always take these medications with food as they can cause an ulcer in a hurry in those with a sensitive stomach. Discontinue taking these and contact your doctor if stomach or gastrointestinal irritation develops. *Consistency* is the key word with both of these treatment modalities. Icing the elbow once every other day and taking anti-inflammatory medications once a day will not have much impact on inflammation. Be more stubborn than the pain!

5. **Stretching**: Stretch 3-5 reps each exercise, holding at least 30 seconds each rep, perform all exercises 1-3 times/day. Stretch to the point of pain and not through it. A long-duration and low-intensity stretch is more effective in lengthening a tendon and muscle than an intense short-duration stretch. Stretching frequently has the added benefit of loading the tendon along its length and pulls gently on its attachment to the bone, thus improving its tensile strength. The trick is not overloading the system by pulling too hard.

Wrist Flexion:

Reach your arm out in front with the elbow straight and palm facing down towards floor, use the other hand on back of wrist and fingers to pull further into flexion, twist the forearmand hand to the outside while holding the palm down, hold 30 seconds. Repeat 3-5 reps.

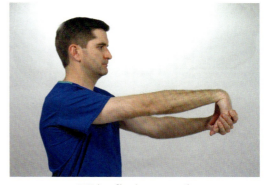

Wrist flexion stretch.

Wrist Extension:

Reach your arm out in front with the elbow straight, lift hand up with palm facing forward, use the other hand to pull back on fingers and palm, hold 30 seconds. Repeat 3-5 reps.

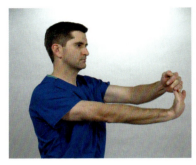

Wrist extension stretch.

6. **Strengthening**: It is easy to overdo strengthening exercises by performing them too early in the recovery cycle. A good rule of thumb is to wait until pain is intermittent before starting these exercises. The elbow should be pain-free while performing these exercises. Adding in one set of reps at a time is another way to sneak into these exercises without causing a bump up of pain and inflammation. For instance, start the first day by performing 1x10 reps. On days 3 through 5, perform 2x10 reps with a 30-second break between sets. Day 6 through 10, perform 3x10 reps with the same 30-second break between sets. When you can perform three sets of 10 with ease and good control, increase to 3x15 reps. When this becomes easy, start to add weight as tolerated. Contrary to the usual American mentality of "more is better", these exercises should only be performed one session per day to avoid causing more inflammation and to allow the muscles and tendons time to recover.

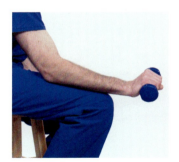

Wrist extension.

Wrist Extension:

Lean forward and place your forearm on thigh with the wrist and hand off the end of knee with palm facing down, grasp a one-pound dumbbell in hand, slowly lift the hand up as far as possible without lifting forearm off of the knee, return down slowly. Follow the same progression listed in the paragraph above. The eventual goal should be to perform 3x15 repetitions, one time per day using an 8- to 10-pound weight.

Wrist Flexion:

Use the same starting position as above, but with the palm facing up. Lift your hand up and down slowly through the available range of motion.

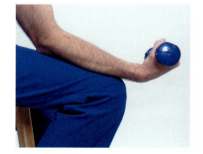

Wrist flexion.

Follow the same progression as described for the first exercise. Goal: 3x15 repetitions, one time per day, using an 8- to 10-pound dumbbell.

Wrist Pronation/Supination:
Place a hammer in your hand with more weight extending above thumb side than below, rotate the wrist slowly to palm-down position, then slowly to palm-up position. Reach farther down the handle to increase the lever arm length as the exercise becomes easier. Progress to a heavier or longer tool as the hammer gets easy. Goal: 3x15 reps, one time per day.

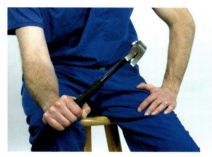

Wrist pronation.

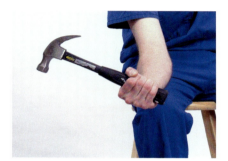

Wrist supination.

Ball Squeeze:
Place a small ball in your hand and squeeze it holding tight for three to five seconds, progress from soft spongel, to a racquetball. Goal: 3x30 repetitions, once a day.

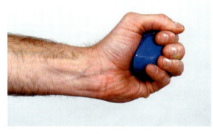

Ball squeeze.

Bodyblade Exercises®
General instructions: Start with continuous motion for 15 seconds and gradually add time towards a goal of 60 seconds. Add a second set to each exercise once you are able to complete all of the listed exercises with good control and no pain. The second set should be progressed from 15 seconds to a goal of 60 seconds in the same gradual manner. Rest at least 15-20 seconds between each exercise. Increase resistance on each exercise as tolerated by moving the blade with more force producing an increased flex in the blade. Refer to page 27 in this book for instructions on ordering a Bodyblade®.

Downward Jab:

Stand with your feet at least shoulder width apart and knees slightly bent for good stability. Grab the handle with one hand so you are looking at the flat edge of the blade. Position your arm down to your side. Move the blade in and out in a jabbing motion. Goal 2x60 seconds.

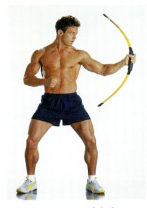

Downward jab.

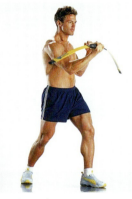

Lunging Upper Cut:

Stand with one foot forward and one back with both knees bent. Grab the handle with one hand so you are looking at the narrow edge of the blade. Move the blade up and down while keeping the elbow bent. Goal 2x60 seconds.

Lunging upper cut.

Chest Press Low:

Stand with your feet at least shoulder width apart and knees slightly bent for good stability. Grab the handle with both hands palms facing down and the flat bladeface towards you. Lower your arms so hands are around waist level. Move the blade forward and backward with a push/pull motion. Goal 2x60 seconds.

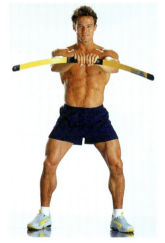

Chest press low.

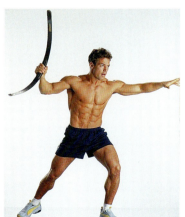

Casting Simulation:

Add this exercise only after all of the exercises mentioned above are well tolerated. Stand with one foot forward and one foot back with knees bent in a casting stance. Grab the handle with one hand so that the thin edge of the blade is

Casting simulation.

pointing towards you. Lift your arm out to the side keeping the elbow bent and hand below shoulder level. Move the blade front to back to simulate the casting motion. Move your arm down and hand in front of your body if this position is painful. (Similar to rubber band external rotation position). Goal 2x60 seconds.

Elbow Program	Date	Date	Date	Date	Date	Date	Date	Date	Date	Date
Wrist Flexion Stretch										
Wrist Extension Stretch										
Wrist Extension Strength										
Wrist Flexion Strength										
Wrist Pronation/ Supination Strength										
Ball Squeeze Strength										
Bodyblade Downward Jab										
Bodyblade Upper Cut										
Bodyblade Chest Press Low										
Bodyblade Casting Simulation										

Make photocopies of this sheet to help you record your progress and stay disciplined with your exercise program.

Use this exercise flow sheet to record the date you performed each exercise. The top half of the sheet contains the name of each stretching exercise and a blank space to record the number of reps performed each day. Example: write in "5x" to indicate that 5 reps were performed.

The bottom half of the sheet contains each of the strengthening exercises with a blank space to record the number of reps and sets performed each day. Example: write "3x10" to indicate that 3 sets of 10 reps were performed. You can record the number of pounds used if dumbbells are used instead of a rubber band. Example: write "3/3x10" to indicate 3 pounds of weight used during 3 sets of 10 reps.

CHAPTER

Wrist Tendonitis and Carpal Tunnel Syndrome

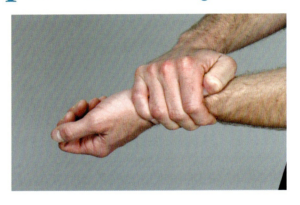

Introduction

W rist pain is a common occurrence in fly-fishermen as described in Dr. Berend's article "Prevalence of Orthopedic Maladies in People Who Fly-fish." His research showed that 12 percent of saltwater fishermen and 31 percent of freshwater fishermen reported wrist pain when fishing. The prospect of increased wrist motion used by the freshwater crowd may account for the higher incidence in this population. In any event, wrist pain is prevalent in fly-fishing, and if left untreated, can disrupt the enjoyment of the sport we know and love.

The wrist joint is much more than just the part of the arm that keeps your watch from falling into the drink. Instead, the wrist functions as the conduit between the motions of the arm and the actions of the hand. To demonstrate the vast motions of the wrist, point your finger at the ceiling. Now, without moving your arm, point to every corner of the room, including those behind you. See, the wrist is truly amazing in its functions. By virtue of our passion for fly-fishing, we anglers put a lot of stress across the wrist.

In order to accomplish the detailed motions and actions that are required of our wrists, we are built with multiple tendons or leaders that originate from the elbow and the forearm. These leaders create not only a great deal of the casting motion, but control the fine detailed actions of the hand and fingers. Furthermore, the majority of wrist ailments originate from these leaders. They must move smoothly in all directions. The leaders are the extensions of the complex muscles of the forearm sending out individual tendons to the top, the bottom, and the sides of the wrist. Individual tendons also extend to the tips of the fingers, over the back of the hand and through the palm.

Not all ailments of the wrist can be blamed on our leaders. Arthritis of the wrist, or more commonly arthritis of the base of the thumb joint, can also cause pain and swelling around the wrist. The information and techniques in this chapter can be used as a general guide to treat or prevent many other wrist complaints which are not specifically named in this chapter.

De Quervain's Tenosynovitis and Carpal Tunnel Syndrome are two common maladies of the wrist. The focus of this chapter was narrowed to these, because they can be so disabling among fishermen.

De Quervain's Tenosynovitis

Symptoms
• A dull ache or soreness at the thumb side of the wrist and forearm.
• Grinding or squeaking sounds may occur during movement of the wrist or thumb.
• Tenderness, burning, swelling, and warmth directly over the thumb side of the wrist and forearm.
• Pain with thumb pinch, hand grasp, or twisting and wringing motions of the hand.
• Pain produced during Finkelstein's test: Place thumb across palm of hand, curl fingers over thumb tightly, move hand sideways away from thumb side. If painful, the condition is most likely De Quervain's Tenosynovitis.

Description

Two tendons from muscles originating in the forearm, *Abductor Pollicis Longus* (APL) and *Extensor Pollicis Brevis* (EPB), run through a small, tight tunnel on the thumb side of the wrist. The tunnel is composed of a fibrous sheath lined by a slippery membrane called the *tenosynovium*. The sheath holds the tendons

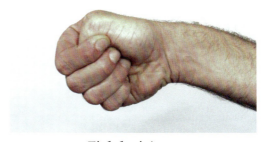

Finkelstein's test.

down so they do not bow out from the wrist. The slippery tenosynovium membrane allows smooth gliding of the tendons within the tunnel. Overuse of these tendons will cause inflammation within the tunnel and subsequent inflammation of the tenosynovium lining.

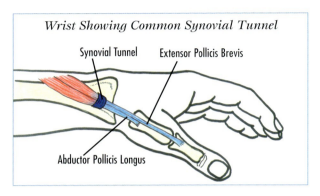

Wrist Showing Common Synovial Tunnel

Carpal Tunnel Syndrome

Symptoms

- Early symptoms: include numbness and tingling on the palm side of the thumb, index (pointer) finger, middle finger, and inner 1/2 of the ring finger, especially upon waking and in the middle of the night.
- Moderate symptoms: ache or shooting pain may occur in the same area described above, or up the arm to the shoulder.
- Severe cases: weakness and atrophy (shrinkage) in the thumb muscles, making it difficult to grasp a cup, magazine, or pencil.
- Pain or tingling reproduced by tapping over the carpal tunnel forcefully (*Tinel sign*), or by closing the tunnel by performing the Phalen's test holding for at least one minute.

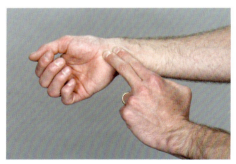

Tinel sign.

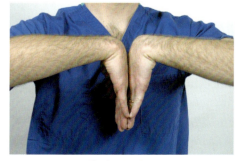

Phalen's sign.

Description

The carpal tunnel is an outlet located on the palm side of the wrist and is formed by a u-shaped basement of carpal bones and a ceiling of ligament (*transverse carpal ligament*). The median nerve and the tendons that flex the fingers occupy this tunnel on their path to the hand. Flexor tendons slide back and forth in this tunnel when you curl your fingers to grasp an object. Much like the tendons that lead to the thumb, as described above, these finger tendons also have a glistening lining of tenosynovium that allows smooth movement. This lining may become inflamed and swollen with heavy, repetitive use. As swelling increases, fluid occupies more space in this relatively stiff tunnel, placing greater pressure on the median nerve and leading to slow nerve conduction or damage. Swelling in the tunnel may also result from any condition that leads to general body fluid retention, such as pregnancy or diabetes.

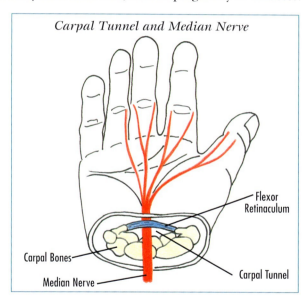

Carpal Tunnel and Median Nerve

Flexor Retinaculum

Carpal Bones

Median Nerve

Carpal Tunnel

General Contributing Factors to Wrist Ailments

A few fishing seasons ago, I (Steve) began the usual quest for rising trout on Montana's Lower Madison River up Bear Trap Canyon. Winter had been unusually cold and long, forbidding the usual midwinter excursions for midge fishing that I have come to rely on for my mental health. This day displayed all the right signs of a successful fish-hunting adventure, including a slight overcast, air temps above 45°, and none of that ungodly wind that routinely assaults the canyon. The canyon road was barren of SUVs and pickups, hinting at few bodies on the river and more of that elusive solitude I was seeking.

> *Rigging my five-weight involved all the usual clumsiness, shaky fingers, and fumbling that comes with the excitement of anticipating fish rising to Baetis on that first spring outing.*

Pulling into the Warm Springs boat ramp further heightened my spirits since only one car and a truck occupied space in "my" parking lot. Rigging my five-weight involved all the usual clumsiness, shaky fingers, and fumbling that comes with the excitement of anticipating fish rising to *Baetis* on that first spring outing. Twisting the tip section onto the butt section resulted in a foreboding twinge of pain in my right wrist. Nothing lingered and I surely wasn't going to let a little pain get between hungry trout and me.

After a brisk walk upstream about a mile and a half, I arrived at one of my favorite gardens of submerged weeds that are home to browns, rainbows, and those pesky white fish. Wading across a small, deep channel brought me to the edge of the weed bed covered in a swirling blanket of currents penetrating its many micro channels in a soothing flow of constant motion.

Studying the surface closely revealed occasional dimples and head forms that betrayed positions of surface feeders eagerly slurping a delicacy unseen for months. False casting until twenty feet of line was free of the reel, I gently laid a reach cast upstream of the largest and most consistent feeder. Slowing my pace and getting in synch with the fish took longer than expected because I was suffering from a long winter of pent-up desire which pumped liberal amounts of adrenaline through my veins. Repeated attempts failed until I slowed my rhythm to match his cold-water cadence. Fish-on!

After slurping my sze18 Hi-Vis parachute Baetis, the silver flash of a 14-inch rainbow coincided with a healthy tug on my rod and was immediately followed by several nice runs and a tail dance. Aching began to override elation as I held the rod high with my right hand while reeling with my left hand. (Why I continue to fish with my reel handle set up on the left-hand side, I'll never know. Change is slow). Landing and releasing the predator revealed the bright red stripe of a spawning male rainbow.

A few dips and splashes in the river removed the slime from my dry fly before blowing most of the water out of its delicate structure. Casting upstream again reminded me of a developing problem in my right wrist. "Override, keep fishing" was the only message that kept coming from my optimistic mind as my body tried to warn of impending peril. Frequent false casting to keep the small fly afloat through the hatch demanded more from my wrist than it was willing to deliver. An ache gradually turned into sharp twinges and escalated to a throb in my inner wrist by the end of that day.

While icing my wrist the following morning, I began to reconstruct the crime scene. My work as a physical therapist had been especially busy for two weeks prior to this fishing adventure and required constant manual therapy to legions of injured skiers, snowboarders, and the customary back-injured Bozemanite hurt by a fall on the icy streets. Hand and wrist fatigue were early signs of system failure that should have been enough to alert me of an impending problem. Because I am first a human being and second a physical therapist, I was able to ignore the early warning signs on Friday and then proceed back to the river on Saturday to inflict more wear and tear on my wrist. End of story. Wrong!

> *That trip exposed me to aggressive surface-feeding fish, one of the most powerful elixirs known to man, and I continued to push on that drug button weekends and evenings to feed the need.*

That trip exposed me to aggressive surface-feeding fish, one of the most powerful elixirs known to man, and I continued to push on that drug button weekends and evenings to feed the need. "I'm a physical therapist, I can stay on top of it with ice and Ibuprofen," was the voice I kept hearing each trip back to the river. After a month of work and fishing, a raging inflammation in my wrist required a week off of fishing, followed by a month of relative rest (for example, 50% less fishing), ice massage, ibuprofen, friction massage, and then exercise before the flare-up subsided. My wrist is now pain-free at rest, but is vulnerable to subsequent flare-ups if good judgment is ignored. The scales had been tipped out of balance resulting in inflammation of the tendon and tenosynovium. I would be thrilled if I could rebalance the scales by working less and fishing more.

Specific Causes of De Quervain's Syndrome

Anatomy

Let's back up a minute and look at how fly-fishing loads these specific tendons. Both of these tendons arise from muscles that originate off the back side of the forearm and travel down to the thumb side of the wrist, pass through the *First Dorsal Tunnel*, and then attach to two thumb bones. One tendon, (*Extensor Pollicis Brevis* EPB), helps to move the thumb into *extension,* which is the plane of motion produced by placing your hand flat on a table with the palm down and moving the thumb away from your hand.

The other tendon (*Abductor Pollicis Longus* APL) is EPB's neighbor in the tunnel and acts to move the thumb into *extension* as described above, or into *abduction*, which is the thumb motion needed to make the hand ready to grasp a large object.

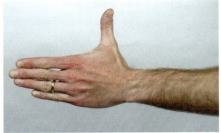

Thumb extension position.

Although each of these tendons produces a specific thumb motion, they can also assist with wrist motion because they cross this joint as well. In medicine, this is referred to as a multi-joint muscle, because it crosses several joints and moves either one of them, depending on how the joints are used.

Fly casting involves a firm grasp of the rod handle with the thumb resting on top of the cork grip. The thumb functions in this position to prevent the rod handle from squirting out of the grasp of the fingers, as well as pushing on the cork to decelerate

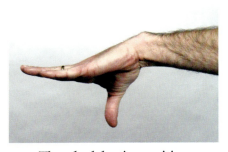

Thumb abduction position.

the back cast, and pushing forward on the cork to accelerate the forward cast. All of these functions are performed primarily by the thumb *flexors,* which are on the opposite side of the thumb from *EPB* and *APL*.

The Thumb Helps Tilt the Bottle

So, how does De Quervain's Tenosynovitis get started in the tendons on the back of the thumb while casting? When the thumb is fixed on the rod handle during casting, the EPB and APL tendons can then perform a secondary movement and assist the wrist into *radial deviation*, which is one of the primary wrist motions needed during casting. Radial deviation is the same plane of motion seen at the wrist when lifting a bottle to the lips, causing the wrist to be tilted towards the thumb side.

So these tendons are dual acting in nature, because they create specific motion at the thumb, and secondarily at the wrist.

> ## *These tendons/muscles contract strongly when decelerating the rod at the end of the forward cast and continue to load during acceleration of the back cast.*

These tendons/muscles contract strongly when decelerating the rod at the end of the forward cast and continue to load during acceleration of the back cast. There is a small amount of *ulnar deviation* (tilting the wrist towards the little finger) motion occurring at the wrist near the end of deceleration of the forward cast, with corresponding *radial deviation* occurring during the acceleration phase of the back cast. This is the same back-and-forth movement produced in the wrist when hammering a nail.

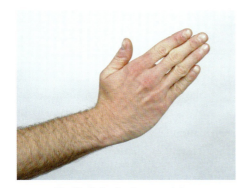

Radial deviation position.

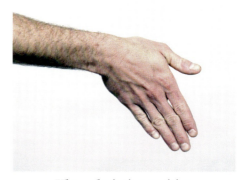

Ulnar deviation position.

Brake Cable Wear and Tear

Overuse in fly casting is the result of placing a tension load through these tendons, while at the same time, forcing the tendons to move back and forth a small distance through their tunnel quickly and repetitively. The tunnel acts as a pulley for the tendons and can break down and become inflamed if too much is thrown at it at once. This is no different than the wear and tear that occurs on a bicycle hand brake cable where it exits the cable guides. The cable is always going to fray and break first at the contact points within the cable guide sheath as it turns towards the brake caliper. The greater the angle change in direction, the more friction force is placed on the cable and its sheath.

Specific Causes of Carpal Tunnel Syndrome

Anatomy

There are other areas of tendon tunnel injury that can develop in the wrist and lead to problems while casting. *Carpal Tunnel Syndrome (CTS)* is a disorder which occurs at the palm side of the wrist where the hand and wrist tendons pass through the carpal tunnel on the way to the hand.

Carpal Tunnel Syndrome is the swelling and inflammation of the tendons where they pass through the carpal tunnel which results in increased pressure within the tunnel, leading to a shut down of the median nerve. Swelling may result from over-use of the hand in poor postures with the wrist extended (for example, typing or fishing), trauma or wrist fracture, and bodily fluid retention disorders. CTS is very rarely caused directly from fly casting alone, but fishing can aggravate an existing condition if it is already present. Fly-fishing requires a strong grasp of the rod by contraction of the flexor muscles, producing a small amount of repeated flexor tendon movement within the tunnel while under load. In its early stages, numbness, tingling, and pain may occur intermittently in the thumb, index, middle, and 1/2 of the ring fingers. As swelling increases and places more pressure on the median nerve, weakness will begin to appear in the thumb muscles making it difficult to pinch or grasp objects. The longer and more consistent that tingling and weakness are present in the thumb, the more likely nerve damage will occur in the median nerve and may eventually become permanent. By the time you're dropping your glass of water two to three times a day, nerve damage is well under way.

> ### By the time
> ### you're dropping your
> ### glass of water two to three times a day,
> ### nerve damage is well under way.

Detecting CTS early is especially important, because nerve damage can be permanent and may result in the functional loss of the thumb's ability to oppose the other four fingers. Try tying on your next Parachute Adams to 5X leader without the use of your thumb and you'll realize the importance of early intervention. See an orthopedic hand specialist or physical therapist early on if nerve symptoms are present, so that appropriate diagnosis and early treatment can possibly prevent more aggressive treatment options.

Casting and Fishing Modifications

De Quervain's Tenosynovitis involves overloading a specific set of tendons as they pass through their tunnel or "pulley". Allowing these tendons to heal requires that you lessen the load that is placed across these tendons while fishing. The previous shoulder and elbow chapters reviewed strategies that can be used to decrease loads to tendons like decreasing fishing frequency and duration, optimizing grip size, decreasing distance from fish, and fishing with a lighter weight rod. A quick review of the information in those first two chapters can help initiate a faster and more complete recovery. These same strategies will benefit the long-rodder when afflicted with a bout of De Quervain's Tenosynovitis or mild Carpal Tunnel Syndrome.

Change is Good

The human body has an amazing ability to adapt quickly to a painful task and find an alternative way to get the job done. A painful low-back injury changes the way you lift a boat anchor off the garage floor. Instead of stooping forward with most of the lifting force and motion coming from your low back, you bend down primarily with your knees performing a squatting motion while the back is kept straight. Pain in one joint automatically causes our body to transfer the motion to a stronger or less painful joint which allows the same function with less pain. When this substitution occurs, the painful joint supplies less of the total motion required and modifies the plane it normally moves in. For example, after an ankle sprain, you find yourself walking with both the foot and leg rotated to the outside more than normal. This allows a rolling motion from the outside to the inside of the foot with each step. Ankle pain in this modified gait is decreased because the ankle joint is not required to bend up and down as far.

Pointer Instead of Hammer

Temporarily modifying joint motion encourages faster healing, because it allows an injured part to rest while completing the original task. The following technique can be consciously employed at the wrist: move the thumb to the side of the cork, then straighten the index finger and place it on top of the grip in the same spot that the thumb used to occupy. Casting in this way uses the rod as a large pointer rather than a hammer.

Another analogy that is commonly used when teaching casting is to use a casting motion that mimics throwing a dart at a dart board. Rather than flinging the dart with a reckless wrist motion, use a steady, constant wrist posture as the dart is thrown at eye level, without much wrist follow-through. This steady wrist posture limits the amount of motion required at the wrist joint, and hence the wrist tendons and finger tendons as well. With these strategies, thumb loading is decreased and the index finger takes over most of the thumb's previous function.

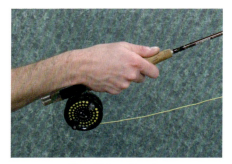

Traditional grip.

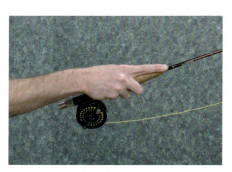

Index finger grip.

Casting with this grip position unloads the thumb and some of its tendons, while increasing accuracy. The index finger is a longer lever arm than the thumb, giving it greater mechanical advantage when applying force to the rod.

> ### *The index finger is a longer lever arm than the thumb, giving it greater mechanical advantage when applying force to the rod.*

Moving the index finger into this position requires that the hand roll slightly towards the thumb side while casting. This transfers load away from the affected wrist tendons in De Quervain's Tenosynovitis (EPB and APL). In this new position, there is less radial/ulnar deviation motion (for example, hammering a nail), and more wrist flexion/extension movement (for example, bouncing a basketball).

I (Steve) have found that changing to this grip has helped me avoid a recurrence of De Quervain's Tenosynovitis, and, at the same time, has increased my casting accuracy at short to medium distances. Longer casts naturally require more outward migration of the shoulder and elbow, making it difficult to keep the index finger on top of the cork at the end of the back cast. If I attempt to cast long distances with the index finger on top, I find myself using the inside of the index finger to push the rod rather than pushing with the finger pad. Not much power there. I quickly change back to a traditional thumb-on-top grip for those longer casts.

Shoot From the Hip

A temporary casting strategy that works well with De Quervain's Tenosynovitis at short to middle distances involves casting with a sidearm motion. Dropping the hand out to the side allows a sidearm casting motion that effectively changes wrist motion from a hammering motion, to a ball-bouncing motion. This effectively diminishes the loading of EPB and APL tendons, because the casting motion transfers more motion to the shoulder and elbow joints while placing less stress to the tendons of De Quervain's syndrome. This casting style should be considered a temporary measure employed long enough to successfully eliminate the original pain, because long-term use can cause painful conditions at the elbow and shoulder. This sidearm cast can be combined with the index finger grip which may further unload the painful tendons and may increase accuracy.

Take a Break With a Brace

Tendon loading can be further diminished by wearing a good-quality wrist splint/brace while fishing or working with the hands. The splint should extend into the palm so that support is given across the wrist joint and lower thumb area. FishermansHealth.com stocks several styles of wrist braces with features that provide the support and features necessary to help control this condition. Other more restrictive wrist braces can be found which incorporate a thumb brace or "spica" into the construction of the wrist brace and further limit thumb motion. Although this can help unload the tendons we've been discussing, the bulk of material in the palm area makes holding the rod difficult for most fishermen. In addition, most of these thumb spicas are fixed with the thumb out to the side in a position that completely restricts the thumb from participating in the grasp of the rod handle.

Get a Grip

Changing the grip of the fly rod to a larger diameter can also off-load the tension required in the tendons that cross the wrist. This is common with golf and tennis, where adjusting the grip size can improve both the power and comfort. The only problem is fly rods don't have big grips. So, the alternative is to wear a comfortable casting glove with build-up in the palm. FishermansHealth.com offers shock and vibration-absorbing gloves in half and full-finger versions that effectively increase the rod grip diameter without having to wrap your beautiful cork with tennis racquet tape.

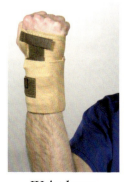

Wrist brace.

In summary, many variables in fishing technique and equipment can be modified to help decrease loads to the tendons of De Quervain's Tenosynovitis and the carpal tunnel. The most productive strategy to initiate early healing involves employing as many of these changes as is reasonable to each fishing situation so that the problem is attacked from many directions at once. Making only one change at a time may not be enough to tip the scales in your favor and promote quick healing.

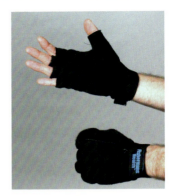

Casting glove.

Treatment

We are not attempting to diagnose or treat any specific ailment, and we encourage you to seek medical attention for any significant complaint you may have that does not respond to self-help care. Furthermore, If you have any numbness and tingling in the hand or wrist, you should probably consult an orthopedic surgeon or physical therapist first to have your condition properly diagnosed and appropriate treatment prescribed. Carpal Tunnel Syndrome includes potential nerve damage and can lead to permanent disability if not treated correctly in the early stages. Treatment of this condition begins with relative rest by splinting the wrist in a neutral position to keep the tunnel as wide open as possible day and night. This condition will require a long period of rest away from grasping, typing, or use of high-vibration tools to allow swelling and inflammation to subside. Other useful, conservative treatments include ice, anti-inflammatory medications, phonophoresis, iontophoresis, stretching of the tendons, or a cortisone injection. If all of these treatments fail, then a surgical release of the tunnel may be required to unload the nerve.

CTS

Treatments 1, 2, 4, and 5 in the section that follows can be safely applied to a suspect wrist with CTS symptoms, as long as the condition shows improvement in three to four weeks. Performing friction massage or strengthening exercises (sections 2 and 5) while CTS symptoms are active may actually worsen the condition and should, therefore, not be performed.

Tenosynovitis

When dealing with De Quervain's Tenosynovitis, the early goal of treatment is to reduce pain and inflammation to the point that it becomes mild and intermittent. Ice, rest, massage, anti-inflammatory medications, and bracing are the early treatment methods of choice when pain is constant and disabling. Once symptoms subside to a lower-level, stretching exercises can be added to the existing program. Gradually progress into strengthening exercises only after most pain has subsided and make sure that none of the strengthening exercises produce soreness during or after an exercise session. Rest is the most neglected aspect of early intervention. You will achieve the fastest recovery if you take a break from fishing and other repetitive activities for one to two weeks while consistently and frequently applying the other treatment techniques. You can use ice and take anti-inflammatory medicine until you're blue in the face, but you will not improve until the tendons are rested! This problem can persist for three weeks to three months, even with consistent treatment and rest.

If all of these self-help, conservative treatment methods fail, you may need to be seen by a physical therapist and receive more intensive treatments like phonophoresis, iontophoresis, manual therapy, or electrical stimulation to help reduce inflammation. If your case is severe, you may need a cortisone injection by your doctor to further reduce inflammation and swelling. The longer you've had the problem, the longer it will take to resolve completely. Some stubborn cases will not respond to cortisone injections and may require a surgical release to fully eliminate pain. Surgery opens up the tunnel and gives the tendons and nerve more room further decreasing friction and inflammation. Follow the program for at least four weeks and continue if you're making progress. If you do not improve, then see your doctor for a more thorough diagnosis and appropriate treatment options. Catch this problem early, and you could save a boatload of time, money, and painful procedures.

> ## Catch this problem early, and you could save a boatload of time, money, and painful procedures.

You can apply all of the following treatment techniques to other types of wrist soreness even if it does not present with the exact set of signs and symptoms as detailed in this chapter.

1. **Rest:** What qualifies as rest? Taking a break from activities that caused the problem is crucial to getting it to go away. If overuse caused the problem, then underuse is part of the cure. Cutting down on the duration and frequency of the offending activity by at least 50 percent is adequate to help mild to moderate

levels of inflammation that have been present for only a short period of time. In severe or long-term cases, rest may mean complete abstinence (a word not commonly used in the American vocabulary) from that activity. Rest allows the body time to repair the injured area by replacing irritating and damaging activities with healing and treatment time. The scales tip in the direction of healing instead of breakdown, and the healing speed increases.

2. **Protection:** A wrist brace provides a secondary form of rest to the inflamed tunnel and tendons. Wrist braces can be purchased locally at your pharmacy or ordered online at FishermansHealth.com. Use a brace long enough to allow other treatment techniques to kick in and reduce inflammation. They should be used daily during activities that stress the hand, but may also be beneficial if left on constantly day and night to keep the wrist and thumb in a neutral position and in complete rest. If you just can't avoid fishing (for example, you're on an expensive week-long fishing trip), then bracing may be your only form of rest. It

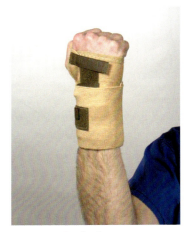

Wrist brace.

must be used consistently to be helpful. Combining the use of a brace with real rest and active treatment is the most effective path to recovery.

Once symptoms are completely absent, you would be wise to use the brace only while you fish the next several weeks to protect the wrist until full strength has returned. Strengthening exercise will ultimately provide the needed healing and stability to the wrist, making the brace unnecessary.

3. **Friction Massage:** Friction massage should be among the first treatment techniques employed to begin stimulating increased blood flow and improve collagen qualities in the tendon. Use several fingertips over the tender area, move the skin back and forth quickly across the tendon in a direction that is perpendicular to the length of the tendon. Perform friction massage to the tendon for 5-10 minutes several times per day. Over the course of several weeks, gradually pushing harder and deeper down into the tendon will provide the best result.

4. **Ice and Anti-Inflammatory Medication:** Reducing inflammation in the tunnel and tendon should be the next treatment technique employed and can be accomplished using ice and anti-inflammatory medications frequently and consistently.

Ice massage should be applied to the painful area of the elbow two to three times per day for about 8-10 minutes each session. Feel the burn!

Ibuprofen or Aleve taken at the maximum dosage listed on the bottle for ten to fourteen days can significantly reduce inflammation levels. Always take these medications with food as they can cause an ulcer in a hurry. Discontinue taking these and contact your doctor if gastrointestinal irritation develops. *Consistency* is the key word with both of these treatments. Icing the wrist once every other day and taking Aleve once a day will not have much impact on inflammation.

5. Stretching: Stretch 3-5 repetitions each exercise, holding at least 30 seconds each rep, and perform all exercises 2-3 times per day. Stretch to the point of pain and not through it. A long-duration and low-intensity stretch is more effective in lengthening a tendon and muscle than is an intense, short stretch. Stretching frequently has the added benefit of loading the tendon along its length, thus improving its tensile strength.

Wrist Flexion:

Reach your arm out in front of you with the elbow straight and palm facing down towards the floor, use the other hand on the back of the wrist and fingers to pull the hand down towards the floor, hold for 30 seconds at the point of pain or stretch. Repeat 3-5 reps.

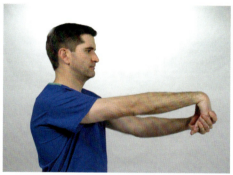

Wrist flexion stretch.

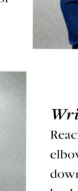

Wrist extension stretch.

Wrist Extension:

Reach your arm out in front with the elbow straight and the palm facing down, use the other hand to pull back on the fingers and palm, hold for 30 seconds at the point of pain or stretch. Repeat 3-5 reps.

Pronation/Supination

Bend your elbow to ninety degrees with arm at your side, open hands and straighten fingers, roll your hand so the palm faces down, then roll the hand so your palm faces up. Repeat slowly up and down holding for 10 seconds at the end of each direction. Repeat 3-5 reps.

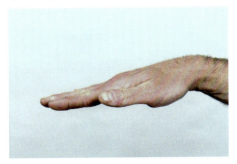

Wrist pronation.

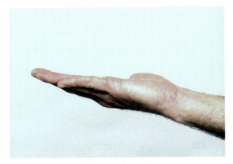

Wrist supination.

Wrist Ulnar Deviation

With your palm towards the floor, place your thumb across the palm and curl your fingers over it, slowly move your hand towards the little-finger side of the wrist, hold 30 seconds at the point of pain. Repeat 3-5 reps.

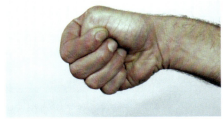

Ulnar deviation and thumb tendon stretch.

5. **Strengthening**: Add strengthening exercises to your program only when the wrist is mostly pain-free with all of the previous exercises. Adding one set of reps at a time is a way to sneak into these exercises without causing a flare-up in inflammation. For instance, start the first day by performing 1x10 reps. Days three through five, perform 2x10 reps with a 30-second break between sets. Days six through ten, perform 3x10 reps with the same 30-second break between sets. When you can perform 3x10 with ease and good control, increase to 3x15 reps. Gradually add weight or resistance once 3x15 reps is well tolerated with a light load. These exercises should only be performed one session per day to avoid causing more inflammation and to allow the muscles and tendons time to adapt. Ice the area immediately after the strengthening session to reduce any inflammation that may have been caused. Many of these exercises can be performed with the use of dumbbells, or modified slightly to use

Theraband®. A six-foot length of Theraband® can be purchased in the blue color at your local physical therapy office.

Wrist Extension:

Lean forward and place your forearm on thigh with wrist off the end of the knee with palm facing down, grasp a dumbbell in hand, slowly lift hand up as far as possible without lifting forearm off of knee, return down slowly. You can substitute Theraband® for a dumbbell weight by standing on one end of the band while in the same position as shown below.

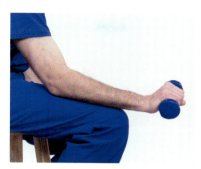
Wrist extension.

Follow the progression listed in the preceding paragraph. The eventual goal should be to perform 3x15 repetitions, one time per day using an 8- to 10-pound weight.

Wrist Flexion:

Use the same starting position as above, but with the palm facing up. Lift hand up and down slowly through the available range of motion. Theraband® can also be used by standing on one end of the band in this same position. Follow the same progression as described for the first exercise. Goal: 3x15 repetitions, one time per day, using 8- to 10-pound dumbbell.

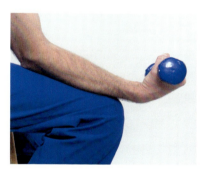
Wrist flexion.

Wrist Pronation/Supination:

Place a hammer or other long-handled object in hand with more weight extending above the thumb side than below, rotate your wrist slowly to palm down position,

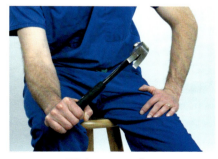
Wrist pronation.

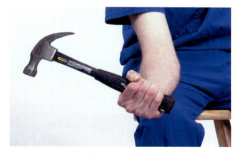
Wrist supination.

then slowly to palm up position. Progress the intensity as tolerated by reaching further down the handle which will increase the length of the lever arm. You may also progress to a heavier/longer tool as the hammer gets easy. Goal: 3x15 repetitions, one time per day.

Wrist Radial Deviation

Grab one end of the Theraband® so that the band drapes over top of fingers and knuckles, stand on the other end, bend your elbow to ninety degrees and hold the elbow stationary while moving wrist up and down. Goal: 3x15 reps., one time per day.

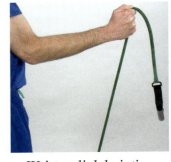

Wrist radial deviation.

Wrist Ulnar Deviation

Tie a small loop in one end of the band and place this loop around a door knob, stand back several feet while facing the door knob, grab the band so that it drapes over top of the fingers/knuckles, reach your arm back with the elbow straight to preload the band, push only the wrist back and forth against tension while keeping the arm still. Goal: 3x15 reps, one time per day.

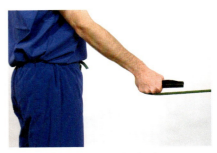

Wrist ulnar deviation.

Bodyblade® Exercises

General instructions: Start with continuous motion for 15 seconds and gradually add time towards a goal of 60 seconds. Add a second set to each exercise once you are able to complete all of the listed exercises with good control and no pain. The second set should be progressed from 15 seconds to a goal of 60 seconds in the same gradual manner. Rest at least 15-20 seconds between each exercise. Increase resistance on each exercise as tolerated by moving the blade with more force producing an increased flex in the blade. Refer to page 27 in this book for information on ordering a Bodyblade®.

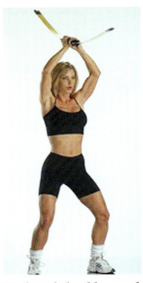

Back and shoulder reach

Back and Shoulder Reach:

Stand with feet at shoulder-width apart for good stability. Grab the handle with both hands so you are looking at the flat edge of the blade. Lift the blade overhead and then produce an up-and-down motion of the blade. Goal 2x60 seconds.

Chest Press Low:

Stand with your feet at least shoulder width apart and knees slightly bent for good stability. Grab the handle with two hands on top, palms facing down and the flat edge of the blade facing towards you. Lower your arms so hands are around waist level. Move the blade forward and backward with a push/pull motion. Goal 2x60 seconds.

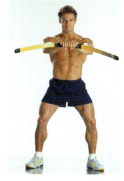

Chest press low.

Tricep Push:

Stand with your feet at least shoulder-width apart and knees slightly bent for good stability. Grab the handle behind your back with a two-hand top grip (same as chest-press grip) with the flat edge of the blade facing up at a 45° angle toward you. Move the blade in a back-and-forth motion towards the floor. Goal 2x60 seconds.

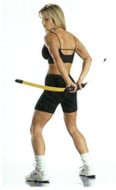

Tricep push.

Casting Simulation:

Add this exercise only after all of the exercises mentioned above are well tolerated. Stand with one foot forward and one foot back with knees bent in a casting stance (you do not need to be in the lunge position shown in the picture). Grab the handle with one hand so that the thin edge of the blade is pointing towards you. Lift your arm out to the side keeping the elbow bent and hand below shoulder level. Move the blade front to back to simulate the casting motion. Move your arm

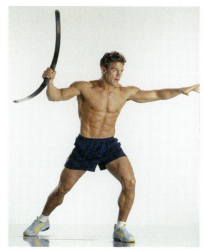

Casting simulation.

down and hand in front of your body if this position is painful. (Similar to rubber band external rotation position.) Goal 2x60 seconds.

Wrist Tendonitis Program	Date	Date	Date	Date	Date	Date	Date	Date	Date	Date
Wrist Flexion Stretch										
Wrist Extension Stretch										
Wrist Pronation/ Supination Stretch										
Wrist Ulnar Deviation Stretch										
Wrist Extension Strength										
Wrist Flexion Strength										
Wrist Pronation/ Supination Strength										
Wrist Radial Deviation Strength										
Wrist Ulnar Deviation Strength										
Bodyblade Back and Shoulder Reach										
Bodyblade Chest Press Low										
Bodyblade Tricep Push										
Bodyblade Casting Simulation										

Make photocopies of this sheet to help you record your progress and stay disciplined with your exercise program.

Use this exercise flow sheet to record the date you performed each exercise. The top half of the sheet contains the name of each stretching exercise and a blank space to record the number of reps performed each day. Example: write in "5x" to indicate that 5 reps were performed.

The bottom half of the sheet contains each of the strengthening exercises with a blank space to record the number of reps and sets performed each day. Example: write "3x10" to indicate that 3 sets of 10 reps were performed. You can record the number of pounds used if dumbbells are used instead of a rubber band. Example: write "3/3x10" to indicate 3 pounds of weight used during 3 sets of 10 reps.

7
CHAPTER

Low-Back Pain

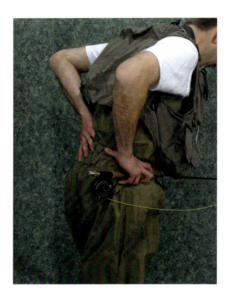

Introduction

Like it or not, at some point in your life, you are likely to have low-back pain. In fact, the medical literature reports that between 66-79 percent of the population will have at least one episode of what we fly-fishermen and women have lovingly termed *stooper's back*. In the Internet-based survey I (Dr. Berend) conducted on the subject, 59 percent of people who fly-fish reported having back pain that they felt was related to their avocation. Additionally, after our first introductory column in *American Angler Magazine*, almost half of the email correspondence from the readers surrounded stories of sore backs, painful wading, and nagging pains in the lumbar spine.

Symptoms
• A dull, constant ache in the middle of the low back that may also spread across the top of the hips to one or both sides and may refer down into the buttocks.

- Intermittent sharp stabbing or pinching pain in the low-back area with bending, twisting, or lifting.
- A catching sensation in the low back on return to erect standing from a forward bent position.
- Increased pain with sustained vertical positions like sitting and standing. Muscle *spasm* (constant painful contraction) of the low-back muscles that can spread up the spine and affect the mid back or even the base of the neck.
- Decreased pain when lying on the back with knees bent, or on one side in a fetal position.

Description

Pain originating in the low back can be caused by overuse of deconditioned *lumbar* muscles that run vertically up each side of the spine, or there may also be pain generated by an underlying inflammation and stiffness in the *facet joints* of the spine. These joints are relatively small and normally help guide the direction each vertebra can move relative to the bone above and below. Tight ligaments, weak muscles, and poor posture may all lead to inflammation of these joints, creating an ache or sharp, catching pain. Both weak trunk muscles and tight hamstring muscles, the strap-like bands along the back of the thighs, can exacerbate a lower back condition. Facet inflammation can eventually progress to arthritis and *stenosis,* or compression of the spinal cord and nerve roots, if left untreated.

Contributing Factors

Wading in the stream or on the shoreline requires constant alterations in the posture of the trunk and legs. Uneven, often slippery ground, strong or changing current, and wave action force the body to constantly adjust to keep from filling those new breathables with cold, spring-run water. It is likely that this constant firing of the postural muscles along the spine causes fatigue and eventual muscular low-back pain. The stooping posture many of us have become accustomed to assuming while trying to be stealth-like in our approach and attack on the trout stream, may also contribute to back complaints. Face it, we abuse our spines and our poor spine's only protection is to be in shape: limber and strong. For some of us, our general conditioning is not up to snuff. That spare tire we carry around is an extra burden on the poor, overworked lumbar spine. So this means conditioning, getting in good shape, strengthening our backs, and stretching those muscles and joints.

> ### *Face it, we abuse our spines and our poor spine's only protection is to be in shape: limber and strong.*

Many other conditions of the spine ultimately result in back pain. Some are trivial in nature, but painful nonetheless. Others can be quite severe and have more serious ramifications if not treated correctly. Low-back pain may also be *referred pain*, originating from an internal organ problem or cancerous growth. So, if you have severe back pain, especially pain that is constant and lasts longer than a few days or is not relieved by rest and a reduction in activity, consult a medical professional before embarking on any new conditioning program. If the exercises at the end of this chapter cause numbness, electric like feelings that shoot down the legs, or undue amounts of pain, you should stop and seek medical attention.

Anatomy

When discussing the causes of low-back pain, it is helpful to go into more detail of spinal anatomy so that a greater understanding can be gained with regards to treatment and prevention of disorders. Our spinal anatomy is an intricate creation of complex mechanical structures with the intermeshing of a delicate nervous system within. The lumbar spine consists of five *vertebrae* at the very lower end of the spine that are stacked one atop the other arising from the foundation bone, or *sacrum*, which is the wedge-shaped bone in the center of the *pelvis*. Each vertebra has a lumbar *disc* above and below that acts as a shock absorber, bony connector, and flexible spacer. The outer rings of the disc are termed the *anulus fibrosus* surrounding the inner gelatinous material containing 90 percent water and are called the *nucleus pulposus*. Facet joints are located on the back side of the spine and are formed by a small, flat bony surface from the bone above and a matching surface from the bone below. They are held together with ligaments called the *joint capsule* and have a smooth, shiny cartilage called *hyaline cartilage* that covers each side of the flat, bony surface. A variety of other strong fibrous *ligaments* connect each vertebra to its neighbor and function to restrict the motion available between each vertebra.

The *spinal cord* contains bundles of nerves, some of which conduct electrical impulses from the brain down the cord to muscles, causing the muscles to contract. Others carry information from the body, for example, pain, hot, and cold, to the brain for input of sensory information. *Nerve roots* are small branches off the spinal cord that exit the spine between each vertebra through a small hole called the

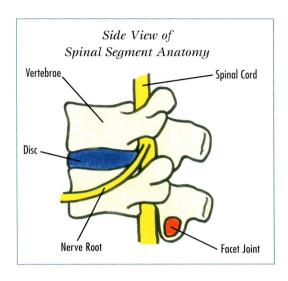

Side View of
Spinal Segment Anatomy

Vertebrae — Spinal Cord

Disc

Nerve Root — Facet Joint

intervertebral foramen formed by a notch in the bone above and a corresponding notch below. These nerve roots are the base of the *peripheral nervous system* and carry messages to and from the brain through smaller and smaller branches throughout the body. Wow, that's a lot of anatomy for one paragraph. It's best to study the illustrations, because they are truly worth a thousand words.

Overlying the back side of the spine are many small muscles that attach from one bone to another and produce straightening and/or rotation of the spine when they contract. In addition to producing motion in the spine, they also reinforce the ligament's role of stabilizing the spine in a vertical posture. In this way, muscles can be viewed as dynamic "guy wires" similar to those seen on tall radio towers that support the structure in a vertical alignment.

> ### In this way, muscles can be viewed as dynamic "guy wires" similar to those seen on tall radio towers that support the structure in a vertical alignment.

Paraspinal muscles run up the back of the spine and assist in extending the spine, that is, return from a stooped position. The *abdominal muscles* are the only muscles that cross the front of the spine. They arise from the front and sides of the pelvis and attach to the front and sides of the rib cage. These "guy wires" up the front side of the tower are critical to vertical spine alignment and also contract when performing a sit-up. If you question the importance of the abdominals, just imagine what would happen to that tall radio tower if one of the support cables was suddenly cut, or like humans, allowed to weaken and stretch out over several years! Cutting a cable is no different than spending hours on the couch protecting those abdominals from any nasty activity or exercise. Eventually they atrophy, or shrink, to the point where they might as well be cut.

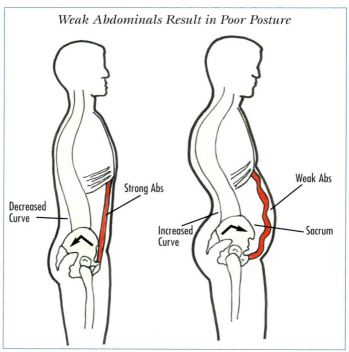

Weak Abdominals Result in Poor Posture

Strong Abs

Decreased Curve

Weak Abs

Increased Curve

Sacrum

Lifestyle

Low-back pain may be generated by any one of these structures acting alone, or more commonly, by a combination of structures weakened over a period of time by a cascade of events. The cascade is usually relatively slow with changes taking place over many months or years, creeping up on the unsuspecting victim. As my friend in Seattle likes to say, "There are no victims, only volunteers." Like it or not, our decisions concerning lifestyle (diet, exercise, posture) play an important role in determining the fate of our low-back health. These lifestyle decisions for us anglers include spending a certain amount of time hunched over, crawling, and hefting our fishing gear or fly vests around the stream. Allowing abdominal muscles to weaken in the years following our last high school gym class is another decision that leads to a cascade into low-back pain.

Gradual Onset

A typical, gradual onset of low-back pain may go something like this: Abdominal muscles gradually weaken over the years with lack of use. Increased abdominal belly fat accompanies lack of use. Both of these conditions lead to an increase of the normal amount of low-back curvature, or *lumbar lordosis*. Belly fat places more weight out in front of the center of gravity and pulls the spine forward. At the same time, weak abdominals can no longer generate enough force to prevent the low back from slumping into an exaggerated curve. Intervertebral discs dehydrate and lose their water content from within the nucleus pulposus causing a collapse in the height of the disc over time. Increased low-back curvature results in the vertebrae tilting backwards on their axis, which decreases the distances between the facet joint surfaces placing them in a state of compression, or *closed packed* position. Closed packed position can be illustrated by looking at the elbow joint in the position of full extension, or straightening. This position takes all of the slack out of the ligaments that cross the joint and thus places the joint surfaces in their most closely aligned and compressed position. Try straightening your elbow and feel how it becomes more rigid and stable in this position. Then bend your elbow and feel how the joint becomes more unstable or lose. Similarly, the closed packed position of the *facet joints* can be found in full extension, or arched low-back position, which places more upper body weight down through the facet joints instead of down through the larger vertebral bodies and discs.

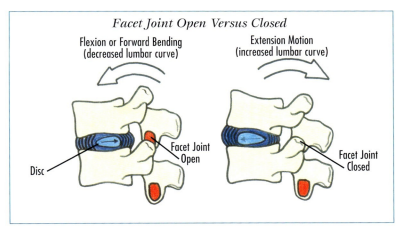

Facet Joint Open Versus Closed

Flexion or Forward Bending
(decreased lumbar curve)

Extension Motion
(increased lumbar curve)

Facet Joint Open

Disc

Facet Joint Closed

Greater weight bearing through the facet joint starts the inflammation process in the cartilage and ligaments of these joints, and over a period of time, initiates osteoarthritis in the smooth hyaline cartilage that covers the surfaces of the facet joints, seen as pitting and bone spur formation of these surfaces.

Listen to Symptoms

Low-back pain includes a wide spectrum of symptoms that lie somewhere along a continuum. If you catch a problem at an early stage, it is easy to halt the progression of degeneration and fully recover relatively quickly. Left untreated, symptoms will increase in intensity and frequency as the degeneration progresses to more and more structures of the spine and leads to permanent and disabling damage. Permanent changes are generally not repairable with conservative treatment or surgery. It's always best to heed the early warning signs beckoning from your low back prior to crossing this threshold.

> *"I know fish are rising now, and won't be rising later in the day, but you better stop casting!" We've all heard that little voice and have become proficient at ignoring it.*

The real challenge is taking the time to listen to your low back pain while in the middle of wading a clear, enticing river or stream. Humans have an amazing potential to deny pain when focused on a pleasurable task and routinely work through intense pain to achieve a desired and pleasurable goal. "I know fish are rising *now*, and won't be rising later in the day, but you better stop casting!" We've all heard that little voice and have become proficient at ignoring it. Pain intensity at these times is often masked or overshadowed by the pleasure of fooling a large brown with a dry fly. What happens when darkness falls and the fish stop rising? From out of the blue the nagging pain emanating from our low back slows our progress back to the truck. But by the time you're telling fish stories the next evening, your pain has backed off and you've forgotten all about pursuing any form of treatment.

Fishing Postures

Most fishing experiences involve standing or sitting for several hours in relative stillness, broken only by short periods of movement over uneven and slippery surfaces. Slide from the truck down the grass bank, slip on the muddy first step into the river, stumble 20-30 yards over greased bowling balls, wrestle across a deep channel, and plant each foot precariously on a river bottom of uncertain elevations. Now stand struggling against a waist-deep, 3-mph current while casting repeatedly for the next forty five minutes. Sit in the drift boat during lunch and on the way to the next hole with the seat too low and your knees up around your chin. Each of these contrasting fishing activities has the potential to irritate the low back when it is in a weakened and deconditioned state. Understanding how these activities can irritate the spine will lead to a better understanding of the need for prevention and treatment techniques.

Wading

Moving over unpredictable and uneven surfaces taxes all parts of the body requiring them to work quickly in concert with each other to produce balanced motion. Even walking on level ground is a miracle in that two small platforms are responsible for stabilizing and propelling a proportionally larger and taller mass forward without toppling. Watching a one-year-old infant walk across the living room floor for the first time illustrates the complexity of a task we often take for granted. *Controlled falling* is the label most often given to walking by those in the biomechanics field when discussing this topic. Each body segment requires a precise firing of muscles crossing each joint to produce enough balanced and coordinated motion in the adjacent segment so that the whole mass is propelled forward at a controlled speed without falling forward to the ground. Throw in an obstacle course of an uncertain river bottom and these same joints need to move through a larger, more unpredictable range of motion in order to adapt to variable footing.

At first glance, walking appears to involve primarily a leg function because legs are the most visible body parts in motion while walking. A second look reveals arm swing, which is counter-directional to the leg motion (right arm moves forward as left leg moves forward). Now we zoom in a third time and begin to pick up a barely perceptible rotation of the spine and pelvis, which allows arm and leg counter-rotation to occur simultaneously. The longer the stride, the greater the spine rotation needed to allow the longer arm and leg swing. A fourth and final look reveals an even more subtle up-and-down motion of the pelvis tilting side to side which is commonly called hip hiking. Faster walking, or walking over uneven ground, forces the pelvis to accommodate motion by tilting further side to side.

So we've started observing motion in the legs and arms and moved to the middle of the trunk to see how the spine and pelvis assist walking. Greater motion occurs in the lumbar spine when walking on uneven rather than level ground. This can lead to overuse or inflammation of the facet joints and surrounding muscles. The greater distance the legs have to adjust while walking over uneven ground, the greater the pelvis and lumbar spine also must move. Demonstrate this on yourself by placing both hands on your hips and feel what happens to the pelvis while walking on even ground followed immediately by walking up stairs. Larger obstacles result in larger pelvis and spine motions.

Size of motion doesn't tell the whole story. Speed and predictability of motion play a large role in determining if walking will become painful to the low back. Have you ever reached the bottom of a flight of stairs and unknowingly stepped off the last two stairs with one large stride? This can be quite a shock to the system, and occasionally painful, because the brain was preparing all your joints for a smaller step instead of the large one taken by mistake. Based on sensory input, our brain constantly predicts needed joint angles, distance of motion, and the amount of muscle contraction needed to move our body smoothly and efficiently. The brain prepares each muscle group to contract the predicted amount necessary to control that particular motion. If the actual motion turns out to be markedly larger than what was prepared for, muscle response is not adequate and results in excessive joint motion to the very end of the range. This is like bottoming out your car on a speed bump because you didn't estimate the size of the bump accurately and hit it faster than the suspension can handle.

Vision makes up a large percentage of the predictive senses that our brain uses to negotiate uneven ground. As you walk in shallow, clear river water, the rocks you see are slightly distorted by the water column and appear larger and in a slightly different location. Increase the water depth, add some silt, and you quickly begin to rely more on *foot braille* techniques than vision to negotiate the section.

> *Increase the water depth, add some silt,*
> *and you quickly begin to rely more on foot braille*
> *techniques than vision to negotiate the section.*

Our brain has a much harder time predicting the next step, and we proceed from one unprepared step to the next, gyrating masterfully to preserve our dignity. No doubt, you've observed how comical it is to watch another angler as he feels his way across an unfamiliar river bottom at full runoff! The lumbar spine and pelvis move through large, jerky motions trying to adapt to unpredictable foot placements with sudden, large weight shifts needed to prevent catastrophe. When we wade all day with the spine working overtime in this manner, low-back pain is a real probability.

Standing and Casting

An even larger percentage of our fishing day might be spent standing still while casting to likely looking water. This is broken only by an occasional step or two to the next fish feeding lane. Even in this relative state of inactivity, postural muscles of the low back and abdomen are constantly firing, adjusting, and balancing our posture. Thus, too little motion can be just as painful as too much motion. A common posture used while casting involves mild to moderate amounts of forward stoop of the upper trunk in the direction that we are targeting. This forward lean is supported by the constant isometric (muscle contraction without motion) contraction of the lumbar paraspinal muscles, which run up and down the spine. Prolonged contraction of any muscle results in an ache in that muscle caused by restriction of blood flow, reduced oxygen, and build up of metabolic waste products. Many of these pain-producing events cause irritation only during the time of the actual contraction, but some may cause residual pain, especially in deconditioned muscles.

This reminds me of my junior high gym teacher who loved to test us by lining us up against the smooth gym wall to see who could last the longest in a 90-degree wall-sit position! Intense burning pain would gradually permeate our quadricep muscles on top of our thighs as we attempted to outlast the thirteen-year-old stud next to us. Something about male competition brings out our greatest effort to endure high degrees of pain for something completely absurd. Throw in a girl's gym class in the same gym, and we could double our personal best. As uncomfortable as the actual test was, nothing compared to the ache and stiffness that followed the next several days as our quads tried to recover and rebuild microscopic damage within the muscle fibers. Change the scenario to that of a huge rainbow sipping midges from the surface film. We rise to the challenge by tripling our most routine efforts and experience muscle overuse and subsequent breakdown pain.

A second form of stationary low-back pain arises when the facet joints of the lumbar spine are positioned in a close-packed or compressed position. Standing increases the pressure across the facet joints, while sitting or squatting opens and removes pressure from the facet joints. Most of us stand with our knees locked straight, an increased arch in our low back, and our waist slightly forward bent. We assume this posture while standing, because our body tends towards the most energy efficient method to get the job done. Or put more bluntly, we're a naturally lazy creature. Locking our knees uses static support from the ligaments, rather than relying on active contraction of the large quad muscles in the front of our thighs which is required in a knee-bent position. Locking our hip and knee joints in full extension while standing places more of the stabilizing loads on the joint capsule and ligaments, and consequently less loads on the energy-consuming muscles.

Unfortunately, lumbar facet joints pay a price for our standing with those lazy leg muscles. Prolonged standing places the facet joints in a close-packed or locked position, increasing wear and tear on the facet joint cartilage. Ache, pressure, and tightness can be felt across the small of the low back after just a few minutes of standing in this arched posture. Pain is produced initially by mechanically overloading the cartilage and ligaments of the facet joint, which stimulates pain-sensing mechanical nerve endings. With time, chemical irritation begins to produce pain caused by the onset of inflammation in those same structures. Those of us with a few more years under our belts notice symptoms more quickly and intensely than our younger counterparts, because we have already developed degenerative changes in our spines and are much lazier in our technique.

> *Those of us with a few more years under our belts notice symptoms more quickly and intensely than our younger counterparts, because we have already developed degenerative changes in our spines and are much lazier in our technique.*

Casting adds a secondary stress to the lumbar spine while standing. A percentage of casting energy and motion are developed through axial rotation (rotation around the long axis) of the entire spine, and can be seen when the upper body twists toward the rod hand on the back cast, and away from the rod hand on the forward cast. This trunk-twisting motion is similar to the mechanics of throwing a ball. In addition, the longer or harder the cast, the more rotation motion must occur in the spine or legs. Forcing the spine to rotate when the knees are locked places most of these twisting loads on relatively small facet joints. Loads on the facet joints can be reduced by bending the knees slightly which allows the knees to twist more freely and contribute more of the rotational force to the cast. This knee-bent posture also changes the low-back curvature which opens and unloads the facet joints.

Sitting

Sitting is yet another stationary position popular to anglers drifting a river or trolling lakes. As with standing, we naturally assume a sitting position that consumes the least amount of energy. A slumped sitting posture with forward rounding of the mid and low back is usually the path of least resistance when we compete with gravity. Other athletes just can't bring themselves to call fishing a sport when much of our time is spent lounging in the bow of a boat enjoying the frothy head from a can of Bud. A case of misdirected jealousy, I guess.

> *Other athletes just can't bring themselves to call fishing a sport when much of our time is spent lounging in the bow of a boat enjoying the frothy head from a can of Bud.*

Seat heights that are too low to the floorboards are common to most small boats, resulting in a slumped low-back posture with knees up around chest level. Low seat positions are often necessitated by narrow, small boat designs in an attempt to keep the center of gravity low so they are less likely to tip over. A slumped sitting posture rounds the low back forward and positions the lumbar spine forward in maximum flexion. Prolonged time in this flexed posture decompresses the facet joints, and increases tension to the back side of the lumbar discs and ligaments. Even a short duration in this posture may result in a general ache or stiffness in the middle of the low back or buttocks. If ignored, further damage can accumulate in the lumbar discs and progress into a full-blown disc herniation.

While in this sitting posture, tension loads are subsequently applied to the back part of the disc's *Annulus Fibrosus* as the disc changes in shape from a symmetrical pancake to more of a wedge shape when viewed from the side. The front of the disc is compressed and the back of the disc expands open, forcing the jelly center (*Nucleus Pulposus*) to migrate back and exert force on the posterior rings (*Annulus Fibrosus)* See illustration on page 93. The inner annular rings begin to break down first resulting in small cracks in these rings and the subsequent migration of gel backwards to the next ring. Gradually, over many weeks or months, more and more rings are fissured progressing from the inside of the disc outward. At some point in the process, a bulge starts to form out the back of the disc causing local pain and may also place pressure on the nearby nerve root.

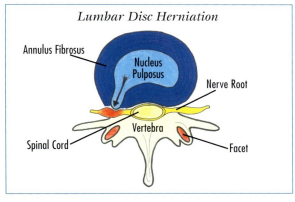

Lumbar Disc Herniation

Annulus Fibrosus
Nucleus Pulposus
Nerve Root
Vertebra
Spinal Cord
Facet

Nerve compression often shows up first as a cramp or ache in the buttock radiating down the outside or back of the thigh, and may be present without any pain in the low back area. Numbness, tingling, and pain may also be present in the lower leg, foot, and toes. This scenario can be more serious than other forms of back pain because prolonged pressure on the nerve root can cause permanent paralysis of leg muscles. Pay attention to the symptoms of leg numbness, tingling, or weakness. Seek early medical help from a physical therapist or spine surgeon if these symptoms are present. The key to success is to catch it early enough to prevent progression to a surgical level. Treatment of a disc herniation is beyond the scope of this book and should be treated under the direct care of a doctor or therapist so that subtle changes can be made to the treatment program as symptoms improve.

Neutral Spine

So, now we have examined the sitting posture, which often places the spine in the opposite extreme of the standing position. It seems like there should be a happy middle ground to this posture issue. And there is! Spine health and comfort are maximized by keeping the spine in a neutral position that is somewhere between the extremes of an excessively arched low back or a position of a forward slumped low back. *Neutral spine* posture evens out the loads placed on the lumbar discs, ligaments, and facet joints by placing them in their most effective and *comfortable* working position. Neutral spine posture can be found in your spine by actively tilting your pelvis back and forth from an extreme arched low-back posture to extreme flat low-back posture. While performing this movement, you will find a position somewhere in the mid range where your spine is the *most* comfortable (this position may not always be completely pain free.) This neutral spine position is unique to your spine and is the optimum posture for your low back whether you are sitting or standing. It takes practice finding and maintaining this posture while out on the water.

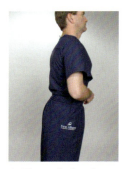

Extended spine.

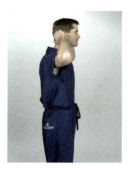

Neutral spine.

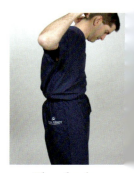

Flexed spine.

Casting and Fishing Modifications

Low-back pain encompasses a vast spectrum of pain intensity and corresponding loss of mobility. Most cases are simply annoying and have only a moderate effect on our fishing adventures. Some cases are extreme and demand that we lie on the floor for hours in agony before we can even think about trying to climb up the furniture to a vertical posture. Common sense goes a long way when we apply the following recommendations to fishing and should win the battle between *cast* or *crash*. Respect your back pain so that you don't "get in over your head" with regards to low-back function while plying the waters. The last place you want to collapse with back spasms is in the middle of a swift current forty feet from the nearest dry land!

Keep it Close to Home

The first variable to consider when in the middle of a bout of low-back pain is the driving distance to your fishing location. Stick close to home for the next several fishing trips and save yourself the trauma caused by a jarring ride as your truck bounces over potholes for miles. Fishing close to home also lets you pack it in and head home if your back hurts. A couple hours of fishing and driving may be all your back can handle while you're in the midst of a severe bout of low back pain.

Your choice of wading and walking conditions is the next variable to consider before heading out the door. Look for a section of river with a smooth gravel bottom, slow current, and a short distance from the car. If deeper and faster water is the only local choice, then use a wading staff to provide that third leg of stability. Avoid fast sections of river and rocky bottoms that challenge even a healthy spine to the max. Bank fishing is an even better idea on those days when unpredictable back spasms strike, making wading a real crapshoot. A little planning will go a long way towards a successful campaign when the low back is flared.

Mix it Up

Success is increased if you plan frequent changes in posture and activities during the course of the day. Most low-back pain is reduced when frequent changes are made every fifteen to twenty minutes and include a mix of sitting, standing, walking, and

Frequently varying your activities keeps the back happy because no one part of the spine is overloaded for too long.

lying down. Lying down on the bank intermittently allows both a change in posture and a relaxation of those fatigued low-back muscles. Frequently varying your activities keeps the back happy because no one part of the spine is overloaded for too long.

The added benefit is that you are forced to cover more good water over the course of a day. Less crowded sections of water allow you to move more often without the fear of losing out on a good hole.

Squat for Relief

Wade to the bank frequently and walk down it to the next promising piece of water. This is easier on your spine than trudging over river bottom through swift currents to the next honey hole. While on dry land, take the opportunity to do the "Third World Fire Squat". Most fishermen with low-back pain or stiffness have probably stumbled on this deep squat position while fishing because it provides a great stretch to tight low-back muscles, and at the same time gaps open the facet joints and decompresses them. You will typically hear an "ahhhh" out of the squatter and may mistake this verbal relief for another bodily function frequently performed in the same position while in the woods. Not to worry, just a fellow back-pain sufferer enjoying a much needed stretch. Researchers have pondered the relative low incidence of back pain in third world countries and have conjectured that squatting on one's heels is far easier on the spine than sitting in a chair. While on dry land, lie down briefly to allow for rest and a change in posture. This is also a great time to perform some of the stretching exercises you'll learn in the treatment section at the end of this chapter.

Cast Creatively

Learning to change fishing and wading tactics while in pain goes a long way towards enjoying an otherwise marginal day. Grab a smaller or lighter rod and move as close to your casting target as possible to reduce the overall size of your casting motion, placing less rotation demand on the spine. Avoid casting large streamers or dry flies as they demand more exertion from the trunk as well. Alternate fishing from the right stream bank to the left stream bank in order to force a change in the casting motion. Utilizing a backhanded motion to flip the line upstream is completely different than standing on the opposite bank and using a forehand motion. Your spine will appreciate the change.

If you are fishing in a rocky stream bed, then place one foot up on a rock to allow that knee and hip to bend. This leg position tilts the pelvis and helps to unload the facet joints in the low back. Change leg positions and place the other foot up on the rock after several minutes to help spread the relief. You may even find that perfect exposed flat rock that serves as a temporary chair from which to sit and cast for a few minutes. Be creative, so you can get your fill of fishing before the low back demands you head home.

Recruit the Whole Body

You can optimize your casting comfort and power by placing the foot opposite your casting arm in a slightly forward position, placing your upper body at a 45-degree angle towards the target. This position allows you to keep your knees bent so they contribute more to the cast while also decompressing the facet joints. In addition to bending your knees, suck in your stomach a little, thereby flattening the curve in the low back and unloading the facet joints even further. Abdominal tightening braces the low back and forces more casting energy to originate from hips, knees, and ankles. Bracing can be assisted using a soft lumbar corset and will be discussed later in this chapter. Remember that neutral spine is defined as the most comfortable position for your low-back and is found somewhere between an overly arched or slumped posture. Neutral spine for a disc herniation is commonly found in a slightly more arched low-back position, because this helps to centralize the disc bulge taking stress off the back of the disc. Neutral spine for a facet joint injury is usually found in a slightly more flexed, or slumped, low-back posture. Spend some time experimenting with your low-back posture to learn the most comfortable position for you. The real challenge is applying this posture on your next fishing trip.

Fishing From a Boat

Many fishing trips involve sitting in a boat for several hours. This places a whole new set of demands on the low back. While sitting looks more comfortable than standing, many low-back conditions are aggravated in this position. The first thing to check is the height of the seat relative to your body size. Optimum seating height allows the hip joints to be positioned slightly higher than the knee joints when sitting in an upright posture. Knees lower than the hips will allow the pelvis to tilt forward slightly, making it easier to maintain some curvature in the low back and achieve neutral spine more easily. Fishermen with long legs tend to suffer more than shorter fishermen because boat seats are extremely low relative to the fisherman's long leg length. This places them in a slumped or flexed low-back posture. Bring along a seat cushion or two on your next trip and place them on top of the seat to help correct the seat height for a better fit. Extra seat cushions can also ease the pounding the spine takes while traveling fast over choppy water in a power-boat. Standing with the knees bent, or bracing with the legs while sitting, may be an even better solution when riding in a fast boat across rough seas.

An alternative seating option involves sitting on the front edge of the seat, dropping one or both knees down, and tucking the feet under the seat. This posture gets the knees lower than the hips and pulls the pelvis forward slightly to allow more curvature in the low back and maintain a neutral spine. Fall back on this technique if you're unable to adjust the seat higher.

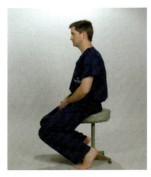

Feet-under-seat sitting posture.

Boat seats with back rests give you the option of leaning against the seat back and letting it support the curvature in your low back. My plastic boat seats are half height and hit me just about mid-back level, providing some degree of contoured support to my low-back curvature. Many fold-down style boat seats are straight-backed rather than contoured and provide little support to the lumbar curve. Place a small, rolled towel, coat, or sweatshirt in the small of your back while sitting in such a seat to provide just the right amount of low-back support. After some experimentation, you should be able to find the perfect roll size for your spine and may even wrap some duct tape around it to maintain the shape for the outing. Of course, you can also buy a full or half-round lumbar support roll from your local medical supply dealer or therapist to achieve the same end result.

Combining several of these seating tactics may be the most effective way to maintain a neutral spine and control pain. Try to adjust the seat height first, then adjust your sitting posture and add the use of a towel roll for back support. Frequent changes in fishing posture gives the low back a break from prolonged static positions and keeps back pain at bay. A good strategy is to change from sitting to standing every twenty to thirty minutes to give your back relief. Many drift boats have knee locks in the bow and stern positions that provide a stable position from which to stand and fish. While standing in the knee locks, tighten your abdominal muscles and keep the knees slightly bent to maintain a neutral spine, provide stable footing, and improve your casting.

Manning the Oars

If you get stuck on the oars for any length of time, make sure to make lots of moaning and grunting noises which will highlight the fact that you're injured and that you probably won't last very long pulling on those oars. Your fishing partner will usually succumb to the guilt of seeing you writhing in pain and let you get back to fishing pretty quickly. Just remember, you can "go to the well" only so many times before it runs dry, so use the drama sparingly. My son Ben has found that he can get out of his "galley slave" duties by navigating my drift boat over a rock or two which then inflicts just enough mental pain on me to force a change in the "rowee" and rower.

> *My son Ben has found that he can get out of his "galley slave" duties by navigating my drift boat over a rock or two which then inflicts just enough mental pain on me to force a change in the "rowee" and "rower."*

In addition to hefting the oars, the man in the middle of the drift boat is usually responsible for pulling up the anchor when leaving that fished-out hole. It's best to stand with the low back slightly arched, stomach tight, and knees bent when hoisting a floor-mounted anchor. (Steve) got lazy (there's that word again) on the Yellowstone while fishing with my son and simply pulled up the anchor with my arms while I was seated. A sudden twinge of pain in my mid back turned quickly into muscle spasm that made breathing or moving a real challenge for several minutes before the symptoms backed off. Fortunately, I had a capable oarsman to take over for the last five miles downstream and a good first-aid kit that included ibuprofen.

In review, look at each fishing situation in light of your painful low back and modify your posture and activities to make your spine most comfortable. If you are fortunate enough not to have low-back pain, adopt these suggestions to assure freedom from low-back pain in the future. Frequent change in postures and activities will always provide the greatest comfort over the course of a day and may even make it more interesting. Apply these changes in combination with the following treatment suggestions, and you will improve the quality of your fishing experience.

Treatment

We are not attempting to diagnose or treat any specific ailment, and we encourage you to seek medical attention for any significant complaint you might have that does not respond to self-help care. Furthermore, if you have any numbness, tingling, or weakness in the leg or foot, you should consult an orthopedic surgeon or physical therapist *first* to have your condition properly diagnosed and appropriate treatment prescribed. This may be a sign of a disc herniation, stenosis, or other more serious conditions requiring additional diagnostics or treatments.

Start with the first four sections of the treatment program below over the course of a week to allow time for your spine to adapt to the new activities, then assess how each stretching exercise is tolerated. Then add the strengthening section gradually as pain allows. If over the course of several days you have increased pain after performing a certain exercise, drop that exercise and move on to others you can tolerate. Slower progress is preferable to moving too quickly. It is normal to experience some increased discomfort during and for a time shortly after some of the exercises, but pain should not linger at this elevated level for more than one hour afterwards. As a general rule, all exercises should be performed at an intensity that causes as little back pain as possible. "No pain, no gain" should *not* be applied in this situation. Go through the motions of each exercise first, and then gradually add more intensity as they are more easily tolerated.

Due to the segmental nature of the spine, hands-on physical therapy treatment can be extremely helpful in freeing up motion in a stubborn joint segment that does not respond to general stretching or strengthening exercises. General stretching exercises may move the vertebrae above and below the joint that is locked, but it may not restore motion to the specific locked joint. Pursuing manual therapy from a skilled therapist can remedy the situation and speed your return to the river.

1. **Protection:** Use of a lumbar corset while performing potentially painful activities is a form of *rest* available to your low back when you don't have the option to completely stop those painful activities. A well-designed lumbar corset may also be beneficial to begin wearing during this painful period. The Fisherman's Health back suport is one such brace with clinically proven technology (www.fisherman-shealth.com).

   Remove the support immediately after each activity to avoid producing progressive weakness in your trunk muscles. Moderate or severe arthritics may find

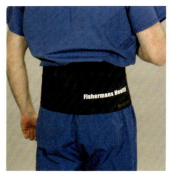

Low back brace open.

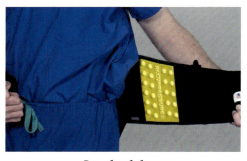

Low back brace.

use of a lumbar support helpful indefinitely while fishing, because it acts second-arily to trap heat in the low back, affording more comfort and ease in motion. There is nothing like an icy cold wind blowing down your stiff and painful low back to stop you cold in your tracks. Corsets will not make you bullet proof and often give people a false sense of security when lifting and bending, so be aware of their limitations. Used wisely, these supports are a great asset for speeding recovery from back pain.

2. **Rest:** When discussing rest with regards to low-back pain, it's important to distin-guish between relative rest and total rest. In the good old days, you were instruct-ed to go home and lie in bed for weeks until your pain subsided. Recent studies suggest that complete bed rest is only beneficial for the first two to three days after acute onset of severe pain or spasms. After that, pain and function will improve more quickly if you get off the couch and walk frequently for short distances. You will also improve more quickly if you avoid any activities or postures that were responsible for bringing on the low-back pain in the first place. This relative rest gives your spine a break from provocative activities, while freeing up time to treat your spine actively.

3. **Heat/Ice:** Muscle spasm often accompanies low-back pain and may wrestle you to the ground in the early stages of an acute flare-up. Contrasting applications of heat for 5-10 minutes, followed by ice for the same duration, repeated 3-4 times each, may get those pesky spasms to relax long enough to allow you to get up off the floor. For this contrasting technique you can use a large bag of frozen peas or corn, and an electric heating pad, hot water bottle, or microwaved rice sock (a large sock filled with uncooked rice, knotted at one end, and microwaved for two to three minutes). Place a small towel between you and the ice pack and lie direct-ly on top of the ice with your knees bent for a comfortable posture. An alterna-tive is to lie on your side, prop the ice bag between you and the back of the couch and insert a pillow between your bent knees.

If you do not have acute spasms, apply heat prior to walking, stretching, and strengthening exercises to relax the muscles and prepare them for motion. Keep the back warm during walking by covering it with an insulator or lumbar corset. Immediately after exercise, lie on an ice pack for 20 minutes, even if you're not in pain at that particular moment. Exercise may increase inflammation levels even though the constant motion of exercise deceptively reduces perceived pain. An hour or two later, pain may increase if you don't ice consistently after each exer-cise session.

The painfully brave may opt for an extreme ice application by enlisting a sadistic spouse or passerby to perform ice massage directly to the afflicted area. Ice massage involves freezing water in a paper cup, and then peeling back the rim to expose one inch of raw ice to be rubbed directly on the skin for 8-10 minutes. Ice massage can be brutal for the first 3-4 minutes, but is ultimately one of the best pain-relieving techniques for the relief of intense pain or spasms.

4. **Walking:** Walking is a critical tool for moving the spine when in pain. The next time you're out walking, place your hands on your low back and feel the muscles contracting back and forth on each side of the spine as you alternate strides. At the same time, feel the pelvis and lumbar spine rotate and side bend with each step. Walking has been shown to be one of the best exercises for the low back at any stage of recovery. Most of us are able to get up and walk indoors for 4-5 minutes even while in the midst of severe back pain. Frequency is more important than intensity when in severe pain, and making that same walk every 1-2 hours during the day will free up motion and decrease pain more quickly. Those with just a dull ache can get outside and start with a 15-minute walk twice a day, and then add 5-10 minutes each day as tolerated, until a goal of one hour is reached. Walk on level, smooth ground and avoid hills or side slopes because they force excessive or unpredictable spinal motion. Distance or time walked is more important than the speed of walking. Hold your abdominal muscles tight while walking so that your low back is positioned vertically, unloading the lumbar spine. Tight abdominal muscles will naturally shorten your stride length and avoid excessive trunk rotation. Keep it comfortable and add time to your walks when your back becomes less painful and can tolerate it.

5. **Stretching**: Flexibility is the next tool in the low-back pain arsenal. Just like any other joint in the body, the lumbar spine generally needs full flexibility to function free of pain. Perform the following stretching exercises immediately after your walk to take advantage of the increased heat and lack of stiffness induced by walking. Use a carpeted floor or pad with plenty of elbow room to provide the perfect back support for these exercises. A couch or bed should only be used if your spine does not allow you to get up and down from the floor easily, because the "give" in these surfaces prevents good feedback to the low back. Move slowly to the point of stretch, stop just shy of pain, then hold for 30 seconds while breathing slowly. Take three slow, deep breaths as an alternative to counting for 30 seconds. Breathing will keep your muscles as relaxed as possible so that the stretch can take the involved joints through their maximum range of motion. Hold the stretch relatively stationary, or move into the stretch further with each exhale as the pain allows, but do *not* bounce at the end range. When in severe pain, start with the

first 2-3 exercises in the list and perform 3-5 repetitions of each exercise. Perform them every 2-3 hours alternating with heat/ice or just ice, until the pain subsides. As resting pain decreases, add the other stretches to your routine until the whole list is tolerated at one session. At that point, you can drop back to 2-3 complete stretching sessions per day. Frequency and duration of stretching are more helpful than increased intensity.

Pelvic Tilt:

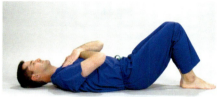

Pelvic tilt.

Lie on your back with knees bent and feet on the floor, suck in your stomach by tightening your abdominal muscles, and at the same time squeeze buttocks together. This should flatten the curve in your low back so that it is touching the floor. Hold for 30 seconds. Repeat five times. This exercise helps to open the facet joints while at the same time teaches control of the lower abdominal muscles. The low-back curve can be monitored by placing your hand under the small of your low back to feel the space between you and the floor.

Single Knee to Chest:

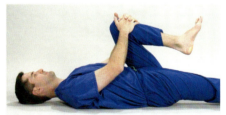

Single knee to chest stretch.

Lie on your back with both knees straight, grab one knee and pull it up towards the shoulder and slightly to the outside until stretch is felt in low back, buttock, or back of thigh. Hold for 30 seconds, and then change to the other leg. Alternate stretching back and forth from one knee to the other until you have performed 3-5 reps on each leg.

Double Knee to Chest:

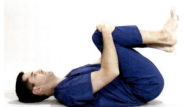

Double knee to chest stretch.

Lie on your back with both knees bent, grab the right knee with the right hand and hold, then grab the left knee with the left hand. Now pull both knees up and out towards the shoulders. Hold for 30 seconds, relax arms to a straight arm position briefly, and repeat stretch 3-5 times. When all reps are completed, return one leg to the floor at a time to ease the strain on your low back.

Rotation:

Lie on your back with one knee straight, bend the opposite knee and place that heel on top of the straight knee, reach the opposite hand to the bent knee and pull it over towards the floor while allowing the spine to twist and hips to roll up off the floor, while at the same time keeping the

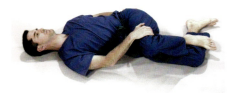

Trunk rotation stretch.

shoulders level. Hold for 20-30 seconds, repeat to the opposite side, alternate back and forth until you complete 3-5 reps on each side. The stretch can be moved up into the spine by bending the lower leg more, and by pulling the upper knee closer towards the chest.

Hamstrings:

Lie on your back with buttocks about 12 inches from the door jam, place one leg through the open door, place the other leg up on the door jam, and straighten the knee. Hold for 30 seconds, and then bend the knee. Repeat 3-5 reps on one leg, then switch to the other side of door to stretch the opposite leg. Slide closer to the door jam if no stretch is felt in back of the thigh, but don't get so close that you cannot keep your hips down on the floor. Do not allow any twisting of the spine. It is normal to get some temporary numbness or

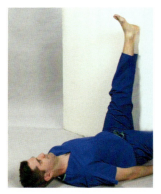

Door jamb hamstring stretch.

tingling in the foot or leg, as long is it leaves as soon as the stretching is finished.

6. **Strengthening**: Good muscle tone is an essential tool to help stabilize the spine in a neutral position while wading, standing, or sitting. As stated earlier, muscles are an important, dynamic stabilizer of the spine and can improve your durability and tolerance of activities such as fishing. Start by adding the first 2-3 of these exercises in the list over the course of one week to allow your spine and muscles a chance to adapt prior to adding additional exercises. Once you are comfortable with the initial exercises at full reps and sets as listed in each exercise, take on the second half of the list. Hold your low back in a neutral spine (comfortable) position while performing all exercises. Neutral spine is the position of maximum comfort for your low back and can be found by moving in and out of a pelvic tilt until that angle of maximum comfort is found. If any of the exercises produce

back pain, back off on the height or distance that you're moving through to see if that will avoid producing pain. Temporarily discontinue any exercise if these changes do not allow you to perform that exercise with minimal discomfort. Add it in a few days later as tolerated. You should perform these exercises once a day as a group to produce the desired fatigue and beneficial strengthening. Start the very first strengthening session with one set of reps, in two days add a second set of reps, add in a third set after another four to five days, or as tolerated.

When all of the exercises are comfortable for the *low back*, increase the intensity of each exercise by following the advice for that specific exercise listed below. Many of these exercises will cause a temporary burn in the muscles being worked no matter how much strength is developed in the muscle. Don't wait for the burning to go away completely in that muscle prior to increasing the intensity of that exercise, because the burning feeling may never change. I guarantee that you will always have an intense burning in the quadriceps muscle on top of your thighs while performing a wall sit no matter how strong and conditioned the muscle is!

Partial Crunch:

A) Straight

Lie on your back with knees bent, cross arms over chest, hold a pelvic tilt postion while lifting upper body off the floor until your shoulder blades clear the floor, hold 3 seconds. This can be made more difficult by clasping your hands behind your neck (support neck with hands only, do *not* pull the head and neck forward), or by holding

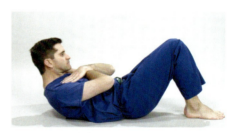

Straight partial crunch.

a weight cuff or plate across chest. Increase reps per set gradually as tolerated. Goal: Total of 3x30 reps (including diagonal reps from exercise below) with 10 pounds of weight.

B) Diagonal

Using the same position as above, lift upper body and twist slightly to one side so that you're looking just to the outside of that knee, hold 3 seconds. This motion should be mixed in with the straight crunches listed above in the following

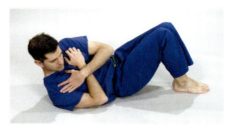

Diagonal partial crunch.

manner: Left, hold 3 seconds, and down; center hold three seconds and down, right hold 3 seconds and down, repeat. Goal: Total of 3x30 reps (including straight reps from exercise above) with 10 pounds of weight.

Prone Arm/Leg Raise:

Lie on your stomach with one or two pillows crosswise under your hips, look straight down at the floor, reach arms up overhead, lift one arm and the opposite leg, just clearing the floor, hold 3 seconds,

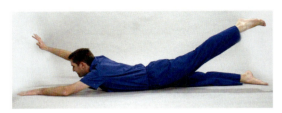

Prone arm/leg raise..

repeat with the other arm and leg combination. Avoid lifting too high (may cause pain in the low back due to hyperextension and rotation). You may start by lifting just one arm or one leg at a time if the combination lift is initially too painful. Add sets and reps gradually. Goal 3x15 reps with 3 pound dumbbells in hands, and/or 3-pound ankle cuff weights on the lower legs.

Unsupported 90°/90° March and Dead Bug:

Lie on your back with knees bent and feet on the floor, perform a pelvic tilt to position of comfort and keep stomach tight, lift one leg up at a time until both legs are in a 90-degree bend at the hips and knees. This is the starting position. Once in this position, lower one leg slowly by moving at the hip joint only (keep knee bent to 90 degrees through the entire move) until the heel touches the floor, return to starting position. Repeat with the other leg until heel touches the floor, return to start. Alternate left and right leg lifts. If this is painful in the low back, then restrict leg movement to a smaller more comfortable range, and avoid touching the floor with the foot. As the exercise gets easier, increase the intensity by straightening the knee, reaching out on each leg movement, and then eventually adding in the arms to perform a full "dead bug". Gradually add sets and reps. Goal: 3x60 reps.

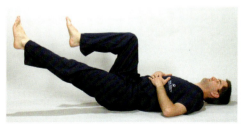

Unsupported 90°/90° march.

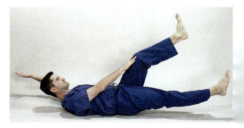

Dead bug.

Superman:

Lie on your stomach with arms reaching out front, lift upper body/arms and both legs up at the same time until they both clear the floor, hold three seconds. Avoid creating pain in the low back by lifting too high off the floor and

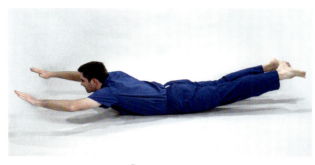

Superman.

hyper extending the spine. Neck discomfort can be minimized by looking straight down at the floor vs. looking forward. Gradually add sets and reps. Goal: three 3x15 reps with 3-pound weights on lower legs and in hands.

Bodyblade® Exercises:

General instructions: Start with continuous motion for 15 seconds and gradually add time towards a goal of 60 seconds. Add a second set to each exercise once you are able to complete all of the listed exercises with good control and no pain. The second set should be progressed from 15 seconds to a goal of 60 seconds in the same gradual manner. Rest at least 15-20 seconds between each exercise. Increase resistance on each exercise as tolerated by moving the blade with more force producing an increased flex in the blade. Refer to page 27 in this book for more information on ordering a Bodyblade®.

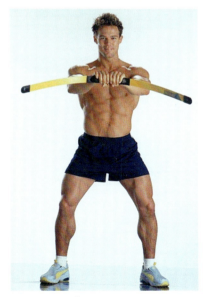

Chest Press:

Stand with your feet at least shoulder-width apart and knees slightly bent for good stability. Grab the handle with both hands palms facing down. Move the blade forward and backward with a push/pull motion to produce a resistance that is challenging in each of the following positions:

A. Arms low with hands at around waist level. (Goal: 2x60 seconds)

B. Arms high with hands at shoulder level, as shown in picture. (Goal: 2x60 seconds)

Chest press.

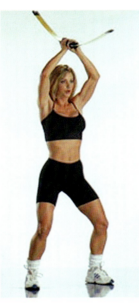

Back and shoulder reach with partial squat.

Back and Shoulder Reach with Partial Squat:

Stand with feet shoulder width apart and knees/hips bent down in a partial squat for good stability. Grab the handle with both hands so you are looking at the flat edge of the blade. Lift the blade overhead and then produce an up and down motion of the blade. Goal 2x60 seconds.

Ab Crunch:

Stand with your feet at least shoulder width apart and knees slightly bent for good stability. Grab the handle with both hands in a two hand top grip, palms facing down looking at the narrow edge of the blade. Move the blade in an up and down motion. Goal 2x60 seconds.

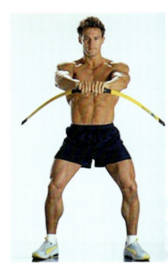

Ab crunch.

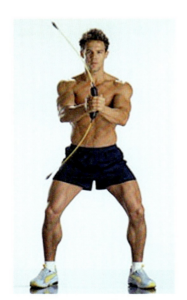

Ab, Hip, and Thigh.

Ab Hip and Thigh:

Stand with your feet at least shoulder-width apart and knees slightly bent for good stability. Grab the handle with all of your fingers interlaced, hold the blade in a vertical position looking at the narrow edge of the blade. Move the blade in a side-to-side motion. Concentrate on holding the stomach tight during the exercise. Goal: 2x60 seconds.

Alternate All 4's:

Begin by assuming a crawling-on-all-4's position. Lift one arm with the Bodyblade up in front of you with the flat edge facing you. Lift the opposite leg out behind you. Move the blade in a front-to-back jabbing motion while keeping your stomach muscles tight and trunk still. Goal: 2x60 seconds.

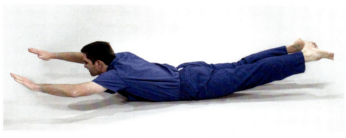

Alternate all 4's.

Conclusion

Our poor backs are the victim of all the terror we place on our body during sport, recreation, and vocation. By virtue of our upright posture, we demand much of this complex structure. It is impressive that 30 percent of us never have back trouble. For the unfortunate, overwhelming majority, lifelong care and conditioning may be the only way to avoid the low back pain hangover that comes after a day on the water.

Low-Back Program	Date	Date	Date	Date	Date	Date	Date	Date	Date	Date	Date	Date
Walking (distance or time)												
Pelvic Tilt												
Single Knee to Chest Stretch												
Double Knee to Chest Stretch												
Rotation Stretch												
Hamstrings Stretch												
Partial Crunch (straight/diagonal)												
Prone Arm Leg Lift Unsupported												
90°/90° March												
Dead Bug												
Superman												
Bodyblade Chest Press												
Bodyblade Back and Shoulder Reach with Squat												
Bodyblade Ab Crunch Bodyblade Ab, Hip, Thigh												
Bodyblade All 4's												

Make photocopies of this sheet to help you record your progress and stay disciplined with your exercise program.

Use this exercise flow sheet to record the date you performed each exercise. The top half of the sheet contains the name of each stretching exercise and a blank space to record the number of reps performed each day. Example: write in "5x" to indicate that 5 reps were performed.

The bottom half of the sheet contains each of the strengthening exercises with a blank space to record the number of reps and sets performed each day. Example:

write "3x10" to indicate that 3 sets of 10 reps were performed. You can record the number of pounds used if dumbbells are used instead of a rubber band. Example: write "3/3x10" to indicate 3 pounds of weight used during 3 sets of 10 reps.

CHAPTER

Knee and Ankle Pain/Instability

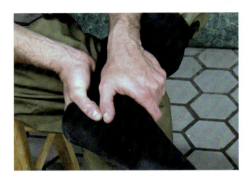

Introduction

Y ou can't catch fish if you can't get to them. This is the type of comment we hear frequently from our patients struggling to return to the sport they love. Lack of mobility prevents our access to the uneven, slippery surfaces that our quarry inhabits. An aging angler is no different than a car rolling down hill. Both are under the powerful tug of gravity which can accelerate their speed if left unchecked. Controlling the speed of a car takes a prudent down-shift and occasional tap on the brakes to slow its descent and prevent a disastrous crash. Similarly, the human body requires frequent exercise and conditioning to slow the effects of aging and maintain our access to the aquatic world.

In this chapter we will discuss some common injuries and degenerative changes of the knee and ankle that can keep us off the water. Joints left untreated tend to progress to a point of instability, pain, and arthritis. Use the suggestions at the end of this chapter to slow your descent towards disability and maintain your access to the fish.

Knee Pain/Instability

Symptoms
• Soreness and pain in the knee accompanied by a sense of instability or buckling.
• Pain is most pronounced while walking over uneven terrain including side slopes,

down hill, down steps, or over slippery surfaces such as snow, mud, or stream bed.
•Tenderness and swelling detected with palpation along the front or sides of the knee joint line.

Description

Knee pain and instability can result from a variety of degenerative conditions and traumatic injuries. Pain and instability may be the result of chronic wear and tear to the knees' *hyaline cartilage*. Hyaline cartilage is the smooth, glistening surface of the joint you see on the end of a chicken bone. Breakdown of this cartilage leads to an arthritic change in the joint surface. These problems usually present as pain and stiffness and become unstable as the arthritis increases.

Traumatic twisting injuries of the knee can produce a greater sense of instability when ligaments or menisci are partially or completely torn. The medial and lateral menisci are the padding cartilage, or shock absorbers, of the knees which provide a cushion within the joint. A medial meniscus tear commonly produces sharp pain or buckling when you walk and may prevent the knee from straightening completely. Meniscus tears are usually painful when squatting deeply or twisting on a bent knee.

Ligaments are stabilizing structures that provide support between the bones of the knee. These can be injured or torn in a forceful fall that takes the joint beyond the restraints of the ligaments. Traumatic tears of the ACL (Anterior Cruciate Ligament) or MCL (Medial Collateral Ligament) may produce severe instability while walking on level ground, or while stepping off a curb.

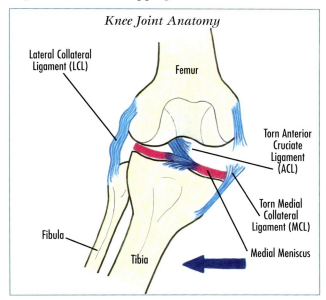

Knee Joint Anatomy

Lateral Collateral Ligament (LCL)

Femur

Torn Anterior Cruciate Ligament (ACL)

Torn Medial Collateral Ligament (MCL)

Fibula

Medial Meniscus

Tibia

Ankle Pain/Instability

Symptoms
- Soreness, swelling, or sharp pain around the outside of the ankle.
- Walking over rough ground or side slopes results in the ankle "giving out" over an inward tilting foot.
- Increased swelling and pain may be more pronounced after activity, or towards the end of the day.
- Pain and instability become more pronounced after each successive re-injury event.

Description
Pain and instability are usually the result of one severe sprain, or a series of repeated inversion sprains (foot rolling in under the ankle) that progressively tears some of the three major ligaments on the outside of the ankle. Most commonly torn is the *Anterior Talo-fibular Ligament,* which crosses the outside front of the ankle and functions to restrict the foot from rolling down and in. Secondly, the *Calcaneal Fibular Ligament* which crosses the outside of the ankle and restricts the rear foot from rolling directly inward. The *Posterior Talo-Fibular Ligament* is less frequently injured, but may be torn with a more forceful inversion injury.

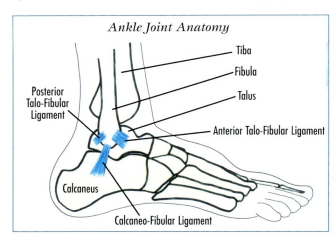

Ankle Joint Anatomy

Posterior Talo-Fibular Ligament

Tiba
Fibula
Talus
Anterior Talo-Fibular Ligament

Calcaneus

Calcaneo-Fibular Ligament

General Contributing Factors
of Both Knee and Ankle Instability

Clamoring along the banks of a Montana river usually requires a good set of legs to negotiate the immense variety of obstacles in one's path. Immediately upon exiting the car our legs are exposed to muddy potholes, barbed wire fencing, and the typical stream access that leads through a narrow gap in cattle fencing to a steep, rocky or muddy bank, sloping down under a bridge abutment. Montana law protects our right to access all public waters at any point where public roads cross rivers, but it doesn't protect our legs from the abuse we face traversing these access points! Although most private landowners have done their best to create a gap between a fence and a bridge or have put in a ladder over the fence, these locations still require agility at the very least, and occasionally the skills of a rock climber to negotiate the access.

If you haven't twisted your knee or ankle after descending through the access, then you have plenty of other opportunities awaiting you as you trek to the first good fishing hole. Heavily fished holes often have a trail beaten through the underbrush that points the way to a proven resource. These established routes have been developed over time by the masses and their tendency to opt for the easiest and most direct route to the river. Much like cattle or deer on game trails, fishermen utilize these proven corridors repeatedly because they contain the least number of natural obstacles between road and river. Some of these established paths may prove treacherous, especially if that stretch of river winds through steep or rocky terrain. It is not uncommon to encounter sizeable rocks, fallen trees, or mud holes along these routes which slow the average rod-toting fish-hunter. Keeping one eye on your rod tip while navigating narrow, overhanging brush can distract your view just long enough to force a stumble over root or river rock.

> *How many times have you fallen hard only to find your rod hand high in the air protecting that precious rod from peril, while exposing your knee, ankle, or wrist to a potential $15,000 surgery and subsequent rehab?*

Geography has placed most streams and rivers at the bottom of steep banks, thus a new set of obstacles materialize as you emerge from the trail and enter the river bank zone. Smoothly-polished river rocks protrude at all angles and heights as you traverse down to water's edge. I find that these sections of our environment often become one of the most common pitfalls to the average knee or ankle. A wrong step on a loose or slippery rock may lead to a quick twist of the ankle or knee while fighting to recover from a devastating fall down the bank, or worse yet, onto your expensive rod. How many times have you fallen hard only to find your rod hand high in the air protecting that precious rod from peril, while exposing your knee, ankle, or wrist to a potential $15,000 surgery and subsequent rehab? "Protect thy rod at any cost" is the automatic fisherman's mantra when negotiating terrain with rod in hand.

Once you arrive at your favorite riffle, entering it safely is the next challenge because of the potential for serious injury. "Look before you leap" comes briefly to mind at this stage in the wading process. As I stand at the edge of a stream my first impulse is to look out over the water to scope for rising fish or likely fish-holding water. Secondly, I evaluate where to step down into the stream. Now, I know what happens if I do happen to be blessed with the sight of a rising trout! The second part of the process often gets ignored, or skipped completely, as my thoughts immediately focus on figuring out what that fish is taking. With eyes fixed on a rising fish, I often stumble off the edge at the closest point of entry, which is usually not the easiest or safest transition point available. Wet grass, slick mud, and loose rocks often conspire to undo my footing as I perform a controlled fall into the water and its immediate river bottom. This is when I usually discover that the water depth is twice my original estimate and that the flat submerged rock is actually round, making that first step an uncontrolled plunge.

Stumbling across slime-covered river rocks to those rising fish is the next test for knees and ankles. Unexpected footing challenges our proprioceptive feedback (the ability of the body to detect joint and limb position) to select stable footing for our advance through the watery terrain. Quick and perpetual adaptation is the name of the game for both knees and ankles while traversing this terrain. Poor water clarity limits our visual input while wading, making it necessary to palpate the river bottom with our numb booted feet while wading in these situations. I often discover deep drop-offs and large boulders by accident while crossing unknown sections of river in the murky spring run-off. Stepping between two rocks often results in a sudden, unpredictable, inward tilting of the foot that can easily end in an ankle sprain.

After hours of casting to rising fish, the end often comes unexpectedly as the hatch tapers off and the fish recede to the depths of the nearest hole. With a smile on my face, I turn towards the bank to take a lunch break and am faced with the task of ascending the river bank. A quick scan of the bank reveals the nearest exit route exhibiting some, if not all, of the most desired characteristics, like shallow water, small first step, gentle sloping bank, good traction, and natural steps in the terrain. As I wade closer to the assumed perfect exit, I realize that the water is deeper than first estimated, making that first step up a real "lulu". Unhindered by this initial realization, I hesitantly attempt this first step anyway, because I know that a change of my plans means wading up or down stream to the next likely spot with no guarantees of a better route. After overcoming the restricted leg movement afforded by my tight waders, I successfully plant that first felt-soled boot atop the bank amid wet grass and mud, which ominously foretells the probabilities of my success. Ignoring common sense and experience, I push up with my elevated foot, only to be surprised when the footing fails, leading to a quick slip and a slam of my knee into a rock jutting out from the slippery dirt bank. On other occasions, rather than a knee slam, my knee folds under as I collapse into a pile on top of that bent twisted leg. Either scenario may produce excruciating pain or embarrassing paralysis as I lie there attempting to ascertain if anyone up or down stream observed my calamity. The second try often invokes unexploited intelligence as I simply place my knee up on the bank first, which shortens my first step and increases my odds of success.

One other potential method of injury and embarrassment that rarely escapes the scrutiny of other anglers is encountered while entering or exiting a boat. Stepping out over the side of a drift boat anchored in a foot of water, tests my flexibility and balance as I make the transition from a moving, elevated surface to a slippery, lower surface. Getting out of the boat mimics the body mechanics needed when an infantry soldier is confronted by an elevated horizontal log barrier when navigating an obstacle course. The best plan of attack involves throwing one leg up over the top while leaning forward and hugging the log on your belly, then rolling over the top and reaching down with a straight leg to feel for the bottom on the other side. The same strategy works when climbing out of a high-sided drift boat. Once the river bottom is encountered, I quickly release the top leg from its perch on the gunwale before the boat moves away from me, forcing the "splits". A more descriptive word could not be found in the English language to describe the visual appearance and bodily experience of such a move. Second only to a groin strain, knee or ankle sprain becomes a definite possibility in this situation due to the combination of an unpredictable landing and a moving boat.

Entering a boat in mid-current can be equally dangerous because the lead leg clamors for footing inside the boat—an unstable surface that moves away with the slightest weight transfer. I have had several graceful entrances in the past while halfway between river bottom and boat, stalling just long enough so that neither surface is adequate to sustain my upright position. I usually find myself hanging from the side of the boat by one leg hooked over the gunwale, while at the same time, hopping along the river bottom with the other foot in an attempt to keep up with the boat now moving quickly away from me. Not a pretty sight.

Specific Causes of Knee Pain/Instability

Now that we have explored many of the situations encountered while fishing that can cause potential injury, let's focus on specific injuries of the knee that can lead to pain and instability. Fishing activities have the potential to produce most of the specific injuries described below, but may likely produce only sufficient forces to cause partial tears of these structures. Other more aggressive contact sports develop far greater forces across the knee, and are more apt to produce a complete rupture of ligaments or tears in the menisci. Whether you've injured your knee while fishing or on the basketball court, a similar mechanism of injury is involved.

The knee joint is a miracle of design in that it is required to move through a large range of motion, while providing stability under severe loads. Huge forces are exerted across the knee because of the extreme length of each bony lever arm extending from its axis. Also, functional activities such as walking, place 100 percent of body weight on only one leg for a very short time. Add the impact load of running, jumping, or hopping, and the forces placed across the knee can exceed 300 percent of body weight! Injuring a knee is similar to breaking a long stick in two pieces. Success is more likely if a large load is applied quickly to one end of the stick while standing on the center of the stick. Application of a large load over a long lever arm in a short period of time produces a large "pop" as the stick, or knee joint, succumbs to the forces. This explains the high incidence of knee ligament injuries in snow skiing, when the long lever arm of a ski places an even greater rotational force across the knee joint.

Knee Anatomy

The knee joint is basically two round balls (the *Femoral Condyles)* sitting on top of a flat table (the *Tibial Plateau).* The ends of each of these bones are covered by a thin layer of smooth, slick *Hyaline Cartilage* which acts to reduce the friction between the two bones. This is the same sort of cartilage as that seen on the ends of a chicken bone: glistening and ultra smooth. Excessive standing, walking over uneven ground, repeated jarring, or poor joint alignment may overload the joint surfaces and provoke abnormal wear of these cartilage surfaces, particularly in people who have other inciting conditions like obesity. It should be noted, however, that many people spend their entire lives standing on concrete at work, running marathons, or playing impact sports without ever having a sign or symptom of knee degeneration. Thus, there is a genetic predisposition that makes a person particularly prone to knee degeneration and arthritis. Abnormal wear leads to arthritic changes within the knee including a thinning, pitting, or erosion of hyaline cartilage with progressive growth of painful bone spurs along the edges of the joint. Intermittent knee pain may progress in severity and frequency, until eventual instability of the knee occurs while walking over uneven surfaces.

Additional shock absorption and stability are provided by the medial and lateral

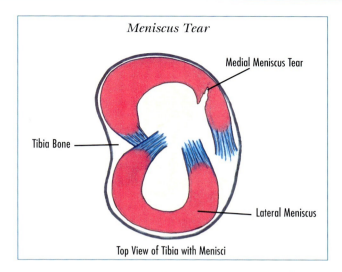

Meniscus located between the *Femoral Condyles* and the *Tibial Plateau*. These quarter-moon-shaped Menisci effectively deepen the joint and provide greater congruency between the flat *Tibia* and round *Femoral Condyles*. They are composed of a slick fibrous cartilage material that acts to attenuate shock and reduce friction between the two bones.

A meniscus can be torn by performing a deep squat, twisting over a fixed foot, or a combination of these motions. This is the classic "torn cartilage" that an athlete would have removed via a lighted surgical microscope called an arthroscope. The resulting flap tear may block available knee motion, produce sharp pain on weight bearing, or promote a sense of knee instability. Very small peripheral tears with minimal symptoms may heal slowly on their own with time and appropriate rehab. Many large, more disabling tears that extend into the center of the meniscus may require surgical intervention. They will not heal on their own due to lack of blood carrying capillaries in the center of the meniscus.

Four distinct ligaments cross the knee joint and function to connect one bone to the other, provide static stability, and restrict end range motion of the knee. The *Medial Collateral Ligament* (or MCL), runs across the medial aspect of the knee joint and functions to restrict knee *Valgus* position ("knock knees"), Tibial *external rotation* (lower leg turned out), and knee *extension* (knee straight). The Medial Collateral Ligament is commonly injured when hit from the outside of the knee by an object or another person in sport, or more commonly in fishing, by falling down while collapsing the knee inward and twisting the foot out at the same time. It is common to tear both the MCL and the *Medial Meniscus* at the same time with this type of fall. Isolated partial tears of just the MCL ligament will heal well with appropriate protection, progression of exercise, and time. They rarely require surgical repair.

Supporting the lateral, or outer, part of the knee is the Lateral Collateral Ligament (LCL). This ligament functions to restrict knee *Varus* position (bow legged), inward Tibial rotation (lower leg turned in), and knee *extension* (knee straight). This ligament is commonly injured when hit from the inside of the knee, or falling with an inward twisting of the lower leg. The LCL is not as frequently injured as the MCL because the mechanisms of injury are less common.

Deep within the knee are two ligaments that cross each other giving rise to the "Cruciate" part of their names. The *Posterior Cruciate Ligament* (PCL) crosses behind the *Anterior Cruciate Ligament* (ACL) to form the cross. The ACL crosses in front of the PCL and functions to restrict lower leg forward translation, internal rotation, and extension. The ACL ligament is frequently injured in cutting and jumping sports, skiing, and awkward falls. The same type of falls that tear the MCL and Medial Meniscus may also tear this ligament, giving rise to the term "Terrible Triad". My neighbor recently tore these three structures while jumping out of the back of his pick-up truck landing hard on both feet collapsing inward on a bent knee. Most people with a torn ACL have a very unstable knee and will require surgical repair to restore functional stability. There are a few rare individuals who can regain stability without surgery, and remain at greater risk of developing a meniscus tear and subsequent arthritis due to greater joint instability.

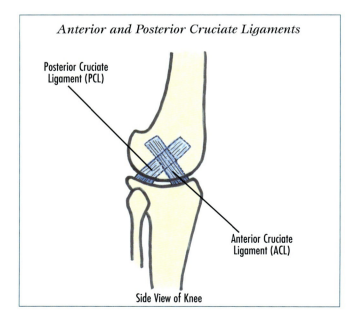

Anterior and Posterior Cruciate Ligaments

Posterior Cruciate
Ligament (PCL)

Anterior Cruciate
Ligament (ACL)

Side View of Knee

The PCL is one of the least commonly torn ligaments of the knee due to the motions that it restricts and the rare combination of events needed to produce this injury. A knee with an isolated rupture of the PCL is rare and usually still quite stable during functional activities. It would be nearly impossible for fishing activities to produce an isolated PCL tear.

> *You are wise to seek an evaluation by an orthopedic surgeon or physical therapist if any of these mechanisms of injury or disabling symptoms sound familiar.*

You are wise to seek an evaluation by an orthopedic surgeon or physical therapist if any of these mechanisms of injury or disabling symptoms sound familiar. After a few days of ice and rest, much of your swelling and pain will decrease enough to allow a good clinical knee evaluation to determine the extent of damage and the next step in treatment. Many of these injuries will require an MRI (Magnetic Resonance Imaging) to look inside the joint and confirm the clinical diagnosis. Old injuries incurred years before may demonstrate similar instability symptoms as an acute injury. These old injuries may respond well to exercise and protection techniques described later in this chapter, especially if this conservative approach was never applied immediately after the original injury.

Specific Causes of Ankle Pain/Instability

Ankle Anatomy

The ankle joint is another one of the body's complex hinges and provides motion in three different planes to allow the foot to adapt to any position while moving over uneven ground, and at the same time, help to propel the body forward. Four distinct bones compose the ankle joint and have many joints between them to allow for this multi-planer motion. The *Tibia* is the larger of the lower leg bones and rests on top of the *Talus*, while at the same time, overlapping the inner side of the talus. Most of the actual weight-bearing force in the ankle is taken through the Tibia resting on the Talus. The Fibula attaches to the outside of the ankle forming a smaller more shallow attachment to the Talus. Most of the motion available at this joint is in a vertical plane and can be seen in sitting when lifting the foot up and down.

Under the Talus lies the *Calcaneus* bone, this is the heel bone. This bone is longer in length from front to back and has a bony prominence on the back for the *Achilles tendon* to attach to it. These two bones form part of the *Subtalar* joint of the rear foot which contributes much of the side-to-side tilting motion needed by the ankle when walking on a side slope. These joints are just like any other joint in the body as they are covered with a thin layer of hyaline cartilage and held together with fibrous bands of connecting ligaments.

Inversion Sprain

Our injury focus will look primarily at the outside of the ankle because it is the most frequently injured area. This is due to the smaller-sized supporting ligaments and greater inversion range of motion available. The typical inversion sprain involves stepping on an uneven surface that forces the bottom of the foot to roll in (inversion) and the ankle to roll out stretching the outer ligaments to the breaking point. The most commonly sprained ligament on the outside of the ankle is the *Anterior Talofibular Ligament* which is at greater risk if the foot is pointing downward at the same time that it is forced inwards. Walking downhill and stepping on a rock may be all it takes to roll the ankle in this way. Skirting down and across a steep river bank is another fishing activity that places the downhill ankle at risk by potentially rolling over an inward tilted foot. The second most commonly torn ligament is the *Calcaneofibular Ligament* which runs vertically up the outside of the ankle and may become sprained with a similar inversion sprain mechanism.

> *The typical inversion sprain involves stepping on an uneven surface that forces the bottom of the foot to roll in (inversion) and the ankle to roll out, stretching the outer ligaments to the breaking point.*

Small partial ligament tears produce immediate pain over the outside of the ankle with some swelling possible after a short period of time and force a slower walking speed over uneven ground. Large tears may be accompanied by the sound or feel of a snap in the ankle, severe pain, extensive swelling, bruising along the outside of the ankle, and leads many people to believe they have broken their ankle. The pop may indicate a complete tear of a ligament, or that the ligament has pulled off a small piece of bone from the fibula. Severe sprains usually prevent further wading and can make walking even on level ground difficult. Any of these sprains should be treated as though they are a broken bone until an x-ray proves otherwise.

Most severe sprains involve complete tears of several ankle ligaments and may require three to four months of rest and rehabilitation, or surgical reconstruction, to regain full stability and function in the ankle. Small partial tears may heal completely with minimal loss of function and allow continued fishing with use of protective brac-ing and exercise. Severe sprains are more disabling because they are so unstable and may lead to repeated spraining events with less and less force needed each time. You are wise to have moderate or severe ankle sprains evaluated early by a professional to determine the extent of injury so that an appropriate treatment plan can be prescribed.

I (Steve) have worked with many older fishermen who have had a history of an old basketball, football, or soccer sprains leading to mild instability and pain while on the water. Many of them have intermittent problems while wading, which are annoy-ing enough to slow them down, but not bad enough to restrict the sport entirely. Many of these folks have never received an adequate evaluation or appropriate exer-cise program following their initial injury. They can benefit from treatment as described later in the chapter. It's surprising how many of these old injuries will improve with a focused exercise program and/or use of an ankle support.

Casting and Fishing and Modifications

Knee or ankle instability can ruin a day, month, or even a year on the water unless appropriate steps are taken to minimize their impact on our favorite pastime. I (Dr. Berend) suffered a severe ankle sprain that was associated with a fracture of the talus bone. This injury required surgery to repair. My point, however, is that some four months later, my ankle feels completely stable except when I'm wading in the stream. Amazingly, the combination of fighting the current, the unpredictable terrain, and the slippery surfaces, makes my ankle feel very unstable. That has forced me to specifically and thoroughly review my equipment to identify changes needed in my current quiver of wading gear. I had no choice but to invest in a very good pair of boots to overcome my ankle instability in the stream. We will now review fishing equipment changes that will help with knee and ankle instability. After that, we'll review use of some supports that can be worn while fishing which will give that shaky limb just enough support so that it doesn't fail you while you're wading. Finally, we will discuss some of the wading, walking, and standing strategies that can minimize the loads on our limbs.

Quality Matters

A good wading boot is worth its weight in gold with regard to fishing success and injury prevention, and is often priced accordingly. In my early days of fly-fishing I (Steve) would hit the year-end sales and pick up the cheapest pair of felt-soled boots I could find, figuring they would only last a short while anyway due to the semi-durable felt soles. I suffered many years as I wore these flimsy, mostly canvas, creations. One year, I splurged on some well-constructed midrange boots and discovered the joys of fake leather supporting my entire foot and ankle. My stability in the river improved, and I found that these higher-priced boots would last somewhat longer than bargain boots.

> *A good wading boot is worth its weight in gold with regard to fishing success and injury prevention, and is often priced accordingly.*

Traction Tricks

Good traction is a real lifesaver when wading streambeds with mossy, slimy rocks. Felt soles are fine for most conditions, but can be improved upon by several modifications that are available commercially. Tungsten studs are finding their way into more felt soles right off the shelf these days and add an additional bite to slime-covered rocks. I have modified felt soles successfully by screwing several 1/4-inch sheet-metal screws into the bottom of the felt soles, spaced every few inches. The screw heads act as cleats digging down through the slime. A recent advertisement in a national fly-fishing magazine promoted a stainless-steel version of these screws, which would probably make them quite a bit more durable than the standard hardware store variety. Additional traction can be gained by strapping on a pair of stream cleats. They have the added benefit of being removable when fishing from the wooden floor of your buddy's drift boat.

My newest pair of boots has interchangeable, multiple soles. This way I can use the excellent support they provide my ankle in all sorts of streambed conditions. Any fly shop worth its retail space will have a good-quality boot that provides ankle support and traction.

Wobbly Waders

Boot-footed waders once the standard attire in fishing, evolved from the early days of fishing with hip-wading boots. These were constructed entirely of rubber and had an integral boot that negated the need for separate boots. However, they were as cumbersome to walk in as a pair of those old rubber rain boots we used as kids. An absence of laces equates to lots of slop of the foot inside the boot with little or no support for the ankle or knee. If you're still wading in a pair of boot-foot waders, then you're due for an upgrade to stocking-foot waders. Your ankle and knee will notice the difference immediately. The extra expense is well worth the safety, support, and pleasure provided by the extra support of a lace-up system. If you're not currently in the market for new waders and are waiting for Christmas or a birthday to roll around, then just purchase an elastic ankle support that is small enough to fit inside your boot-foot waders. These can be found online at www.fishermanshealth.com. Orvis now makes a pair of waders with lace-up boots attached, giving one more option to the wading world.

A Third Leg

Deep, fast rivers may require the added stability gained by a third leg. Don't rush out and look for a pair of waders with three legs, just purchase a collapsible wading staff that can be worn in a holster on your wading belt until needed. This third leg can be used downstream of your body while crossing fast or deep water, providing extra stability and a little more time for your next foot placement. It can also be used as a hiking staff when walking the trail to your next fishing hole or descending a steep bank.

Sleeves For Stability

Mild knee instability can be decreased by wearing a neoprene sleeve over the knee inside your waders. Some sleeves have a hole cut out of the front for the knee cap and may include Velcro straps to add additional compression and stability. They assist the knee by retaining body heat, controlling knee-cap motion, and most importantly, by providing proprioceptive feedback so the knee becomes more stable. The sleeve will not prevent dangerous motions from occurring, but it will forewarn your body when you're moving into a vulnerable position, enabling your body to fire the appropriate muscles automatically to avoid buckling. Pressure and tactile sensory stimulation increase in intensity as your knee bends or twists inside the sleeve, creating a proprioceptive feedback loop to the muscles and resulting in more accurate control of the joint.

> *Pressure and tactile sensory stimulation increase in intensity as your knee bends or twists inside the sleeve, creating a proprioceptive feedback loop to the muscles and resulting in more accurate control of the joint.*

The sleeve should fit snug enough to place some compression on the knee, but not so tight that it restricts circulation. When sizing a sleeve, you should be able to get two or three fingers up under the sleeve without having to stretch the fabric significantly when the knee is straight.

Severe forms of knee instability may require the use of a hinged neoprene or fabric sleeve with extension stops built into the hinges. These usually have built-in metal stays extending up the medial and lateral sides of the joint and provide a little extra support to a knee that tends to hyperextend or collapse inwards. These hinged braces are a small step up in the level of support provided as compared to a plain sleeve, but may be more bulky and uncomfortable due to the additional hinges and stays. I would seriously recommend getting an orthopedic consultation from a knee specialist prior to purchasing this higher level of support. If you feel a need for this higher level of support, you may already have enough knee damage to warrant surgery.

The same can be said for an ankle that remains unstable after the completion of a strengthening and balance training exercise program along with the use of a compression sleeve. Several over-the-counter braces use lacing, stays, or stirrups up the sides of the ankle to restrict ankle inversion motion. Many of these braces do a great job of preventing lateral instability, while allowing the normal up-and-down motion needed in forward walking. Because bulk is a problem, fitting these braces inside your wading boots may require that you sacrifice that extra pair of socks to allow it all to happen. A flexible fabric lace-up with removable stays or stirrups may give you the flexibility needed to adjust the brace to your particular needs. I (Dr. Berend) was unable to wear these complex ankle braces under my stocking-foot waders, so I upgraded to a better pair of boots and continued to wear a lightweight ankle support that provides some level of compression and the proprioceptive feedback as described above. These ankle sleeves are available on-line at www.fishermanshealth .com.

It Comes From the Sole

Ankle and knee stability can both be improved by adding foot orthotics (custom-shaped insoles to modify foot and ankle position) inside your waders. These devices are usually custom-made by a podiatrist from a plaster cast of your foot, and are built to correct for structural foot and ankle problems. Ankle pronation is a common problem that can be caused by abnormal foot structure which results in a flat-foot walking position and subsequent knock-kneed position. Correcting this alignment problem through the use of orthotics can improve knee and ankle stability, while at the same time, decreasing joint pain. Proper use of foot orthotics requires a firm, close-fitting boot with a stable heel counter (cup around heel) to control motion. Using one without the other is ineffective.

Wading and, Walking Strategies

Once you have taken inventory of your wading equipment and made the necessary changes, it's time to move on to wading and fishing tactics that can make or break your next trip. You can control many variables while fishing that will have a large impact on your knees and ankles. The more painful or unstable your joints are, the more seriously you should look at controlling these variables in order to protect the joints from greater injury.

A little planning of your next outing goes a long way towards tailoring your fishing around the level of function your painful joint is capable of tolerating. Let's face it, most of our fishing adventures are driven by where the fishing is currently hot rather than where the easiest wading is located. June in Montana can deliver an amazing salmonfly hatch on both the Yellowstone or Big Hole rivers, but not as good on the Gallatin or Missouri rivers. Armed with this knowledge, while being bombarded with first-hand stories of big fish devouring dry flies, I'm naturally drawn to the most productive waters.

> *Now, I'm not advocating complete denial of the salmonfly hatch, just a little selective planning to keep it pleasurable, painless, and productive.*

Now, I'm not advocating complete denial of the salmonfly hatch, just a little selective planning to keep it pleasurable, painless, and productive. Pick a section of river in the desired location with easy access from the road, smooth walking surfaces, and slower current to help make your day more enjoyable. To further reduce stress to the injured joint, keep wading to a minimum by mooching a ride in a friend's drift boat for the day. After all, salmonfly imitations are usually more effective when thrown from the middle of the river towards the bank.

Seasonality of fishing determines the change in location of current hot fishing spots and changes in the environmental factors that influence walking and wading ease. Local winter fishing can be amazing when the air temps rise above 40 degrees for a few days and the midge hatch lures fish to the surface for some protein hoarding. Difficulties arise when attempting to walk along the edge of river-bank shelf ice that has suddenly turned from a rough, frozen solid to a slick, wet surface, making each step an impending scene from the Three Stooges. In addition to becoming slick, ice also becomes weaker and collapses underfoot in these warmer temperatures, resulting in a sudden drop of one leg through the ice to the river bottom. Pick your spots wisely and look at them with an eye towards accessibility rather than pure fish-catching potential.

Winter also has a tendency to layer freestone river banks with several inches of snow, providing just the right amount of slickness to degrade one's traction. There are days while walking up or down river when I feel as though I've survived running the tire drill in football practice as the snow-covered rocks have similarly challenged my agility and balance. Dealing with snow-covered rocks is only half the challenge of winter walking. Snow tends to build up on the bottom of felt soles growing to two or three inches thick, and producing the sensation that you're walking on croquet balls strapped to the bottom of your feet. Some of the newer rubber-soled wading boots can help prevent some of this snow buildup while plying the banks.

Think twice about where you're headed during this time of year and plan to fish known sections of rivers that do not require a long walk to the first hole or the need to traverse steep and rocky banks. Accepting a small compromise in fishing location may allow you to get outside safely and fish a day that would have otherwise been lost to the couch.

Treatment

We are not attempting to diagnose or treat any specific ailment, and we encourage you to seek medical attention for any significant complaint you may have that does not respond to self-help care. Consult a doctor or therapist prior to starting any of these exercises if you have suffered a painful injury where you also heard or felt a corresponding pop in the joint, as you may need additional diagnostics or surgery prior to starting any exercise. Furthermore, cases of severe pain, instability, locking, or catching should always be evaluated by a doctor or therapist first to rule out serious injury requiring surgery. In addition, if you have any numbness, tingling, or weakness in the leg or foot, you should consult an orthopedic surgeon or physical therapist first to have your condition properly diagnosed and appropriate treatment prescribed. This may be a sign of a lumbar disc herniation, spinal stenosis, or other more serious condition requiring alternative treatment.

Recent traumatic injuries with residual joint swelling or discoloration should be treated more cautiously and the exercises progressed more gradually to allow the soft tissues time to adapt while healing. Pushing exercise too aggressively immediately after injury may overload the soft tissues and prevent them from healing correctly. Use of joint-protection braces and taking a rest from aggravating activities are critical to the normal healing of a sprained ankle or knee ligament. A healing ligament may heal in a slack or stretched-out position if it is not protected for the first eight to twelve weeks. During this time, restrict the size of the motions used while exercising. For example, when recovering from a typical inversion ankle sprain, avoid stretching or strengthening the ankle into painful end range inversion (foot turned in), as this could overload the injured ligaments and cause them to heal loosely.

Try adding only one or two new exercises each day to the program because they are more easily tolerated. If an exercise produces pain in the joint and lasts for more than an hour after exercise, that exercise should be eliminated temporarily or cut back in intensity and repetitions until it is tolerated more easily. Instead of forcing a painful exercise, move on to other exercises and then attempt a few reps of that difficult exercise intermittently to determine when it will be tolerated more easily. Pain does not mean gain, despite the teachings of my old high school coach.

> *Persistence pays off with most rehab programs as functional gains improve slowly over time with a gradual increase in intensity and duration.*

Persistence pays off with most rehab programs as functional gains improve slowly over time with a gradual increase in intensity and duration. On the other hand, if you are *not* making some progress after performing the exercise program over several weeks, then quit and seek help.

1. **Protection**: Most painful and unstable joint problems benefit from the use of a brace to help protect the joint from overloading the healing ligaments while exercising. In addition, they will improve proprioceptive feedback during functional tasks and improve balance. Most flexible braces provide additional compression to the joint to help reduce swelling. The brace

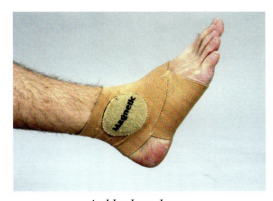

Ankle sleeve brace.

should be used while fishing or walking on uneven ground. Take the brace off when indoors, on level ground, while lying down, and while sleeping. Use of any brace full time may lead to muscle weakness or prevent circulation to the foot and toes, thereby slowing the healing process.

Ankle sleeves may be purchased at your local drug store, sporting goods store, or online at Fishermanshealth.com. Knee sleeves and hinged braces can also be found at most drug stores, and sporting goods stores.

2. **Rest**: Most acute sprains will heal more quickly if you provide relative rest to the injured leg by avoiding painful activities. If it hurts to walk or stand for more than thirty minutes, then limit your activity time to below that threshold until pain and swelling improve. Gradually decrease rest and increase exercise as pain and swelling allow.

3. **Ice and Anti-inflammatoryMedications:** Reducing inflammation and swelling in the acutely sprained joint can be accomplished by using ice and anti-inflammatory medications frequently and consistently for the first 10-14 days after injury. Apply ice packs over a thin hand towel that covers the skin. Use an ace bandage wrapped over the top of the ice pack to hold it in place and provide some compression to the joint for swelling control. Leave the ice on for 15-20 minutes, and use it at least 3-5 times per day. Take at least an hour break between icings. Older injuries can benefit from applying an ice pack once a day immediately after exercises or at the end of the day.

Any of the non steroidal anti-inflammatory medications like Ibuprofen or Aleve can be taken on a regular basis after injury and may assist in the reduction of inflammation. Take these medications at the dosages indicated on the bottle and keep them in your system day and night for the first 10-14 days after an injury. Take them with food to prevent the risk of developing gastro-intestinal (GI) problems. Discontinue them immediately and contact your doctor if you develop a sour stomach, pain, or other GI discomfort.

4. **Massage and Elevation:** Most acute knee and ankle injuries will develop some joint swelling that can impede healing if left untreated. Swelling can be decreased early on by lying down and elevating the injured leg on pillows making sure that it is above the level of your heart. The leg should be elevated as long as possible during the first seven to ten days after injury. As pain allows, bribe your spouse or pay a professional to massage your leg while it is elevated, working from the foot up towards the body which will help pump the excess fluids out of the leg while increasing local blood flow to the area.

Start performing friction massage across the injured ligament for five minutes, one to two times a day, starting about seven days after injury, or as soon as tolerated. This will help the ligament heal faster and stronger as is outlined in the earlier treatment chapter.

5. **Stretching**: Begin stretching the injured joint up and down to help regain the lost

bending and straightening motion. Avoid stretching a freshly injured joint in a side-to-side plane, or with a twisting force, because this motion may cause the ligament to heal loosely, or not at all. Perform all stretching exercises 3-5 reps, 2-3 times per day.

Ankle

Ankle Dorsiflexion/Gastroc Stretch:

Stand facing the wall with the injured foot back and the good foot forward. Keep the injured knee fully extended, bend the good knee, lean forward until a stretch is felt across the front of the ankle, calf, or both. Do not allow the heel to lift off the floor. Hold for 30 seconds, repeat 3-5 reps.

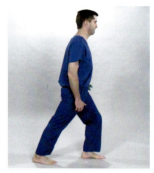

Gastroc and ankle stretch.

Ankle Dorsiflexion/Soleus Stretch:

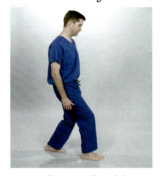

Stand in the same position as above, with the exception of moving the injured rear foot forward until the toes are almost touching the good heel, squat down bending both knees and ankles until a stretch is felt in the front of the ankle, back of the calf, or both. Do not allow the heel to rise up off the floor. Hold for 30 seconds. Repeat 3-5 reps.

Soleus and ankle stretch.

Knee

Hamstring/Knee Stretch:

Lie down on floor with injured heel resting on the door-jamb and knee straight. Place the other leg through the open door with knee straight. Slide as close to the doorjamb as possible while still keeping hips and buttocks on the floor. Hold 30 seconds, repeat 3-5 reps. As the muscle relaxes, move closer towards the doorjamb. It is normal to experience some temporary numbness and tingling in the foot.

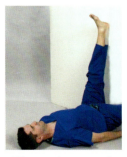

Hamstring stretch.

Quadriceps/Knee Stretch

Lie on your side with the injured leg on top, bend lower knee up towards chest, grab upper leg at ankle and pull thigh and knee back behind you. Hold 30 seconds, repeat 3-5 reps.

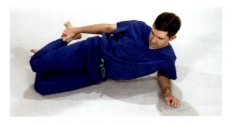

Quad and knee flexion stretch.

6. **Stationary Biking:** Ride a stationary bike with a light tension adjustment. This allows the joint to move with very little body weight and encourages the production of *synovial fluid* inside the joint that acts as a lubricant and brings nutrition to the cartilage. Biking also improves strength and range of motion in a stiff joint. An early ankle sprain may tolerate this activity more easily by placing the middle of the foot on the pedal, rather than pushing through the ball of the foot. Start with 5-10 minutes at a slow-to-moderate speed, then add time and speed as tolerated. Goal 20-30 minutes.

7. **Strengthening Exercise**: The following exercises benefit both knee and ankle pain/instability problems and can be added slowly to your exercise routine (2-3 exercises at a time) to ensure a gradual progression and to sort out the exercises that may be problematic early on. For fresh ankle or knee sprains, start these 7-10 days after the injury and follow the specific advice listed in each exercise concerning acute injuries. It is normal to experience some local stiffness and soreness while performing these exercises. Those exercises that produce sharp pain, catching, locking, excessive grinding, or joint popping correlated with a sharp pain, should be avoided. You may be able to come back to the problematic exercise in several weeks and perform it without these symptoms occurring. Stop exercising and see your orthopedic doctor or physical therapist if these symptoms do not improve during the first two to three weeks. These exercises should be performed once daily and ice should be applied afterwards as described earlier in this chapter.

Ankle

Heel Lifts:

Stand facing a countertop and place one finger from each hand on top for balance, place feet about eight inches apart with feet pointing forward, push up onto balls of feet as high as pain allows. Start with 3 x 10 reps and gradually increase to 3 x 20 as tolerated, progress to hanging heels off the back of a stair step, then to performing while standing on one leg.

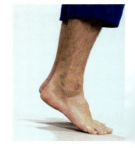

Heel lifts.

Toe Lifts:

Stand facing a countertop, place feet about eight inches apart, lift forefoot as high as pain allows. Start with 3x10 reps and gradually increase to 3x15 as tolerated, progress to one leg as tolerated. This is a smaller-sized muscle group than the calf muscle and fatigues more quickly with fewer reps.

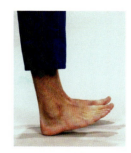

Toe lifts.

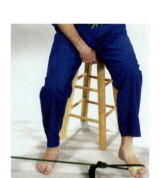

Band eversion exercise.

Rubber-band Ankle Eversion:

Sit in a chair with knee bent to about 80 degrees, loop band around forefoot (best done with shoes on) so that the band is perpendicular to the leg, push foot out and up against band while pivoting on heel. The other end of the band can be secured around a table leg, or knotted and passed through the hinged side of a closed door. Start with 3x10 reps and gradually increase to 3x20 reps as tolerated. At that point, add tension to band by moving away from door, or by sticking both feet through loop and pushing both feet apart at once. Bands can be purchased at your local physical therapy office.

Rubber-Band Ankle Inversion:

Start in the same position as in the eversion exercise, but with band at the opposite side, push foot inward and up while pivoting on heel, avoid painful end range motion by keeping the movement relatively small at first. Start with 3x10 reps and gradually increase to 3x20 reps as tolerated. Then add more tension by pre stretching the band.

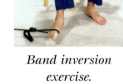

Band inversion exercise.

The Alphabet Game:

Sitting or standing on one foot, use the big toe to draw each letter of the alphabet. Gradually and purposefully spell out every upper case letter: A, B, C... By the time you get to Z, the foot and ankle experience positions they have never been in before. This adds strength, agility, and proprioceptive feedback to the ankle. Alternate this exercise from one ankle to the other.

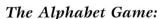

Alphabet game.

The Towel Game:

Standing on one foot, use the other foot to pick up a hand towel off the floor. Lift the towel to your hand without bending forward at the waist to grab it. This takes practice, but once you have the small muscle coordination and strength, increase the effort and skill required by using larger towels. Alternate this exercise from one ankle to the other. If you can pick up a beach towel, I would bet you are unlikely to suffer from foot and ankle problems on the water.

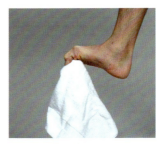

Towel game.

Knee

The Straight-Leg Raise:

Lie flat on your back on the floor or workout bench. Completely straighten one leg. Bend the other leg up with the foot flat on the floor or bench. Now raise the straight leg about 6 inches off the ground. Hold the leg in this position with the knee straight for a one count. Now, bend the knee slowly, lowering the foot to the ground. Once the heel touches the ground, straighten the leg again, holding it 6 inches in the air. Hold for a one count then lower the entire leg to the ground. Once you have the rhythm, it should flow: lift-one, bend-two, straighten-three, and down-four. I usually say these words to keep the timing correct. This exercise works the quadriceps muscle group in the front of the thigh. It also targets the patellar tendon that runs from the knee-cap to the front of the shin. Start with 3x10 reps. Add ankle weights to increase tension, goal of five to ten pounds.

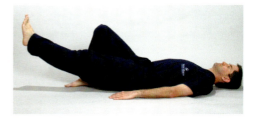

Supine straight leg raise exercise.

Forward Step Up:

Stand facing a regular stairstep, place the injured leg on the step and leave it stationary during the entire exercise. Step up *slowly*, then step the uninjured foot back down *slowly*. Start with 3x10 reps and gradually increase to 3x20 as tolerated. At that point, increase the intensity by making the step height taller (add books to the top of the stair, step up to

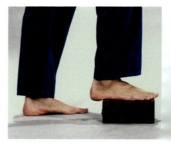

Forward step up exercise.

fireplace hearth, find a sturdy box, or the seat of a sturdy chair). The goal is to increase step height so that the thigh is parallel to the floor in the starting position (knee bent at 90-degree angle). If you have to jump up, or drop down, then the step is too high.

Forward Step-Down:

Stand on top of a phonebook with both feet, step off the front edge with the *uninjured leg,* and touch the heel to the floor, return slowly to the top of the book. Repeat 3x10 reps and gradually increase to 3x20 as tolerated. Increase the size of the step by stacking more books and progress by 1- to 2-inch increments as tolerated towards a goal of 6-8 inches high. Always use a step height that allows full motion in a controlled manner without

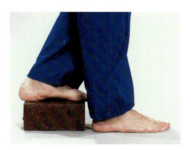

Forward step-down exercise.

knee pain. Always keep the knee centered over the second toe and prevent it from collapsing inwards (prevent a knock-kneed position)

Wall Sit:

Stand with your back to the wall, step each foot out front about 10-12 inches (shoes on for traction), slide your back down the wall until the knees are bent to 90 degrees or above knee pain, hold for 10 seconds. Start with 3x10 reps and gradually increase the hold time to 30 seconds. If knee pain is present, stop slightly higher up the wall at first. It is normal to feel a burning ache in the quad muscles in this position no matter how strong you get!

8. Ankle and Knee Balance/Proprioceptive Training: These exercises can be performed for either knee or ankle instability and will help improve balance and strength. Perform these exercises with shoes on to support the arch in the foot and provide a solid platform to the foot and ankle.

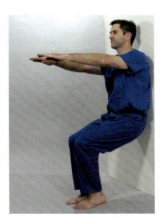

Wall sit exercise.

Rubber Band Kicks:

Place the loop around your *uninjured* ankle, step back so that all of the slack is out of the band, lock both knees straight and stand on one leg, kick the uninjured leg in a front-to-back direction through about 10 inches of motion as quickly as possible without letting either knee bend (kick from the hip, not from the knee). Start with 3x15 kicks in each of the following directions.

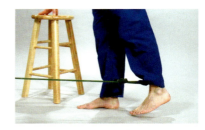

Theraband® kick exercise.

A. Facing the band attachment point.
B. Facing away from the attachment point.
C. Standing sideways to the attachment point (leg with band is closest to attachment) The direction of the kicking motion is always in the same front-to-back direction despite the different band positions. The exercise should be progressed by adding a little more tension to the band, and later on by standing on a foam pad or folded towel.

Rubber Band Abduction Steps:

Place loop around uninjured ankle, stand with injured hip towards the attachment point and all of the slack out of the band. Lift foot up and then step *slowly* out to the side about 2 feet and place that foot on the ground in a wide squat position, then return that same foot *slowly* back next to the other foot. Start with 3x10 reps and gradually increase the size of the step

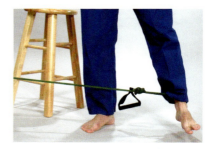

Abduction step exercise.

and the tension on the band for greater challenge. Balance and strength are challenged by always moving *slowly* side to side.

Rubber Band Adduction Step:

Turn so that the non-injured side is facing to the attachment point, start in a wide-squat stance with all of the slack out of the band, step the uninjured foot *slowly* placing it alongside the other foot, return *slowly* to a wide-squat stance. Start with 3x10 reps and make it more challenging by stepping out in front (heel to toe) of the fixed foot, then make it even more difficult by stepping completely over the top of the fixed foot. Tension can also be added. *Slow* is always better than fast.

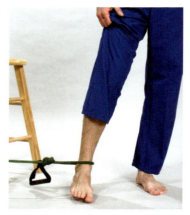

Adduction step exercise.

Bodyblade® Exercises

General instructions: Start with continuous motion for 15 seconds and gradually add time towards a goal of 60 seconds. Add a second set to each exercise once you are able to complete all of the listed exercises with good control and no pain. The second set should be progressed from 15 seconds to a goal of 60 seconds in the same gradual manner. Rest at least 15-20 seconds between each exercise. Increase resistance on each exercise as tolerated by moving the blade with more force producing an increased flex in the blade. Refer to page 27 of this book for information on how to order a Bodyblade®.

One Leg Standing Balance:

Grab the handle with the hand on the same side of the body as the leg you are standing on. Have the narrow edge of the blade facing you. Stand on the injured leg with knee bent and lift the other foot up off the floor. Move the blade in an up-and-down motion. Goal 2x60 seconds.

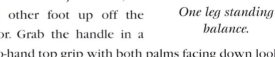

One leg standing balance.

Chest Press Standing On One Leg:

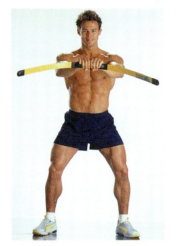

Stand on the injured foot, lift the other foot up off the floor. Grab the handle in a two-hand top grip with both palms facing down looking at the flat edge of the blade. Move the blade forward and backward with a push/pull motion. Goal 2x60 seconds.

Chest press standing on one leg.

Jab Standing On One Leg:

Stand on the injured foot, lift the other foot up off the floor. Grab the blade with the hand on the opposite side of your body from the leg you are standing on. Keep the flat blade face towards you. Lift your arm out to the side and move the blade in and out in a jabbing motion. Goal 2x60 seconds.

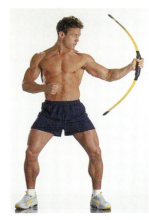

Jab standing on one leg.

Ab, Hip, and Thigh

Stand with your feet at least shoulder width apart and knees bent in a partial squat for good stability. Grab the handle with the fingers of both hands interlaced, hold the blade in a vertical position with the narrow edge of the blade towards you. Move the blade in a side-to-side motion. Concentrate on holding the stomach tight during the exercise. Progress to standing on one leg when this gets easy. Goal 2x60 seconds.

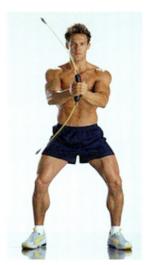

Ab, hip and thigh.

Keeping a leg up on the knees and ankles can be the difference between a beautiful day on the water and a day spent falling, sliding, slipping, and mostly cussing your way down the river. The complexity of these joints makes them very susceptible to injury, instability, and painful degenerative conditions. Performing stretching, strengthening, and proprioceptive feedback exercises will literally help you keep your legs beneath you while fishing.

Ankle Program

Ankle Program	Date	Date	Date	Date	Date	Date	Date	Date	Date	Date
Bike (time or distance)										
Ankle Dorsiflexion/ Gastroc Stretch										
Ankle Dorsiflexion/ Soleus Stretch										
Heel Lifts										
Toe Lifts										
Band Eversion										
Band Inversion										
Alphabet Game										
Towel Game										
Band Kicks (front, back, side)										
Band Abduction Step										
Band Adduction Step										
Bodyblade One Leg Standing Balance										
Bodyblade Chest Press Standing on One Leg										
Bodyblade Jab Standing on One Leg										
Bodyblade Ab, Hip and Thigh										

Make photocopies of this sheet to help you record your progress and stay disciplined with your exercise program. Use this exercise flow sheet to record the date you performed each exercise. The top half of the sheet contains the name of each stretching exercise and a blank space to record the number of reps performed each day. Example: write in "5x" to indicate that 5 reps were performed.

The bottom half of the sheet contains each of the strengthening exercises with a blank space to record the number of reps and sets performed each day. Example: write "3x10" to indicate that 3 sets of 10 reps were performed. You can record the number of pounds used if dumbbells are used instead of a rubber band. Example: write "3/3x10" to indicate 3 pounds of weight used during 3 sets of 10 reps.

Knee Program

Knee Program	Date	Date	Date	Date	Date	Date	Date	Date	Date	Date	Date
Bike											
Hamstring/Knee Stretch											
Quad/Knee Stretch											
Straight Leg Raise											
Forward Step Up											
Forward Step Down											
Wall Sit											
Rubber Band Kicks (front, side, back)											
Band Abduction Step											
Band Adduction Step											
Bodyblade One Leg Standing Balance											
Bodyblade Chest Press Standing on One Leg											
Bodyblade Jab Standing on One Leg											
Bodyblade Ab, Hip and Thigh											

Make photocopies of this sheet to help you record your progress and stay disciplined with your exercise program.

Use this exercise flow sheet to record the date you performed each exercise. The top half of the sheet contains the name of each stretching exercise and a blank space to record the number of reps performed each day. Example: write in "5x" to indicate that 5 reps were performed.

The bottom half of the sheet contains each of the strengthening exercises with a blank space to record the number of reps and sets performed each day. Example: write "3x10" to indicate that 3 sets of 10 reps were performed. You can record the number of pounds used if dumbbells are used instead of a rubber band. Example: write "3/3x10" to indicate 3 pounds of weight used during 3 sets of 10 reps.

9
CHAPTER

Last Cast

When the last rise has evaporated into tiny rings and ripples, and the only insects left are doing more biting than being bit, the angler leaves the stream to journey back to the car. Many of us spend countless hours preparing for that day on the water. We tie innumerable patterns, many of which, if you're like me, will never get wet, let alone set into the jaw of a weary trout. But we plan, tie, plan, scout, plan, and fish as much as possible. We spend hours in the local fly shop, spinning yarns of fish that get bigger and adventures that are now much more exciting than when they were actually etched into our minds. It is this reflection on the day's events and the seasons of fishing that keeps the angler motivated to head out again. The memories and photographs of big fish and small hold us till the next time we can don the waders and fling the weight-forward into the pool.

In the chapters of this book, we hope to have spawned a similar preparation and reflection on conditioning, stretching, and strengthening for our sport: fly-fishing. I was once given a necktie that showed a cartoon-like picture of two men, both overweight and deconditioned, coming to the revelation that if fishing is sport, they too must be athletes. This is true. Among us are many who spend time on the links or the courts chasing a small white ball or a larger yellow ball. Why should golf and tennis be sports with athletes the likes of Tiger Woods and Andre Agassi, and not fly-fishing with Lefty and Flip? Fishing is a sport with its own set of stresses and injuries. Like golf and tennis, our elbows and shoulders will show signs and symptoms of overuse and poor conditioning.

If these ailments are so common, why not do something about it? That is where Steve and I came together. With a foundation of decades of flyfishing experience, Steve's expertise in physical therapy, and my knowledge of musculoskeletal problems, we teamed together to develop the first book devoted to preventing and treating the problems so common to men and women who call the stream home.

This book outlined a series of exercises and modalities directed at treating or preventing the common problems identified in my scientific study. But reading is only the first, and least important, step towards ridding yourself of the demon that is musculoskeletal pain. The bigger and more vital component is doing it! Programming yourself to do the exercises on a regular basis, stretching in and out of season, and learning about the cast and how it affects your body are the important parts. Next time you pick up a book or magazine article on casting techniques, look past the how-to and investigate what stresses the motion is placing on the wrist, elbow, and shoulder. While surfing Saturday morning TV observe how the heavy vest and poor posture might affect the low back after a day of fishing. Learn to identify the stresses that fishing can place on our bodies and do something about it. Face it, we are going to fish, fish as much as humanly possible, but conditioning, stretching, and strengthening will get us through it with less pain and discomfort.

We have only dimpled the surface on the lake of understanding when it comes to fly-fishing. Little is known about the human body and its needs when casting the long rod. Research has clearly defined the detailed mechanics of the baseball pitch and has calculated that the shoulder joint needs about 130 degrees of eternal rotation flexibility to safely pitch in the major leagues. How much external rotation does the shoulder require to safely cast 60 feet of line to bonefish all day? No one knows. There is much to learn about the sport we love.

Glossary

Abdominal Muscles

A group of muscles in the lower trunk composed of several deep and superficial muscle layers acting to produce trunk flexion and rotation motion as well as stabilize the spine.

ACL (Anterior Cruciate Ligament)

A ligament located deep in the middle of the knee which helps restrict forward motion of the Tibia under the Femur, Tibial external rotation, and hyperextension of the knee. It is frequently torn in skiing, or cutting and jumping sports.

Anterior Talo-fibular Ligament

A ligament located on the outside-front of the ankle which helps restrict the foot from rolling in under the ankle. It is frequently sprained with an inversion ankle injury.

Achilles tendon

A large tendon in the back of the ankle which is a connection from the calf muscles to the back of the heel. Frequently inflamed or torn in cutting and jumping sports.

Acromion

A bony prominence jutting off the top of the shoulder blade which deepens the shoulder socket. It can be a frequent site of impingement on the rotator cuff depending on its shape and size.

Acute

Term used to describe an injury that is either very recent or intense in nature.

Aleve

Name branded medication composed of Naproxen Sodium which is a NSAID (Non-Steroidal Anti-Inflammatory Drug) acting to decrease inflammation and pain.

Annulus Fibrosus

A dense fibrous material making up the outer ring layers of a spinal disc. It is frequently torn in a disc herniation.

Arthritis

The gradual erosion of the smooth hyaline cartilage layer covering the inside of joints.

Axial Rotation

A term used to describe the twisting motion of a bone, limb, or trunk around its long axis.

Bodyblade®

A patented exercise device consisting of a flexible shaft with a handle in the center and small weights on each end.

Brace

A external structure applied around the outside of an injured joint used to restrict motion and prevent re-injury.

Bursa

A thin soft tissue sack with slippery fluid inside that is common throughout the body in areas of potential friction between tendons and bones. It reduces friction forces between structures by gliding upon itself like a water balloon pressed flat on a table.

Buttocks

The term used to describe the anatomical area of the rear end which is composed of the Gluteus Maximus, Gluteus Medius, and Gluteus Minimus muscles.

Biceps Tendon

This usually refers to the tendon connecting to the long head of the Biceps muscle in the upper arm. The tendon is frequently involved in Impingement Syndrome as it becomes irritated by excessive friction forces under the Acromian bone.

Bruise

Discoloration of the skin due to trauma and subsequent rupture of capillaries in the area.

Buckling

A term used to describe the sudden forward collapse of the knee while walking due to instability after injury.

Bursitis

Inflammation and swelling of a Bursa due to overuse and excessive friction forces across the bursa.

Calcaneus

A bone located in the bottom and back side of the foot commonly referred to as the heel bone.

Calcaneal Fibular Ligament

A ligament located on the outside-back of the ankle which helps restrict the foot from rolling in under the ankle, or the Fibula sheering forward on the Calcaneus. It is frequently sprained with an inversion ankle injury.

Capillaries

The smallest branch of blood vessels which transports blood to the body at a cellular level.

Clavicle

The bone across the front of the upper chest commonly referred to as the "collar bone". It attaches to the Acromian bone of the scapula to form the AC joint.

Collagen

A type of soft tissue fiber that is a microscopic component of all connective tissues like tendons and ligaments.

Contrasting Hot/Cold

Repetitive applications of alternating heat and cold to an injured body part to help reduce swelling, increase circulation, reduce muscle spasm, and reduce pain.

Cellular

A reference to anatomy or physiology functions which occur at the smallest structural level.

Chronic

A term used to describe pain that is long standing in nature.

Close-packed

That position of a joint at which the capsule and ligaments are at maximum tension, surfaces are most congruent, and joint compression forces at there highest.

Common Flexor Tendon

The tendon which attaches several different forearm flexor muscles to the Medial Epicondyle of the inner elbow.

Compression

Use of an external elastic wrap to apply circumferential pressure to an injured body part for the prevention and reduction of swelling.

Deconditioned

A term used to describe a general state of fitness which is inadequate to support a full level of function.

Deltoid muscle

A muscle that covers the outer aspect of the shoulder joint which functions to lift the arm away from the side.

Elastin

A specific type of connective tissue normally found in tendons, ligaments, and fascia which provides the property of elasticity.

Elevated

To place an injured body part in a position that is vertically higher than the level of the heart to promote the drainage of fluids out of the limb.

Eustachian tube

A tube in the female anatomy which connects the ovaries to the uterus and functions to transport a fertilized egg to the uterus.

Extensor Carpi Radialis Brevis

The muscle originating from the out side of the elbow and extending across the back of the wrist. The contraction of this muscle produces wrist extension, or backward bending of the wrist.

External Rotation

A term used to describe rotation motion of a bone or limb away from the midline of the body.

Eversion

A term used to describe motion of the ankle in an outward direction.

Facet joint

A joint on the back side of the spine formed between two vertebrae, existing in pairs, one left and one right sided. This can be a site of pain generation due to compression forces and the development of inflammation.

Femoral Condyles

The rounded shapes at the lower end of the femur bone which form the upper half of the knee joint.

Fibula

The smaller of two bones in the outer aspect of the lower leg and forms the lateral aspect of the ankle joint.

Fibrosis

Microscopic changes frequently seen in injured or overused tendons with resulting scar tissue build up and thickening of the structure.

Finger Extension

A term used to describe finger motion as seen when the hand is opened vs. closed.

Foot Orthotics

Custom made insoles that are manufactured from a cast of the foot. They are designed to correct bony/structural deformities in the foot and ankle to improve function and decrease pain.

GI

An abbreviation used for Gastro-intestinal.

Golfer's elbow

A slang term used to describe pain and inflammation of the common flexor tendon at the inner aspect of the elbow.

Hamstring muscle

A group of three muscles running down the back of the thigh and across the back of the knee which bends the knee and straightens the hip while walking.

Humerus

This bone is the single bone in the upper arm.

Hyaline cartilage

A smooth shiny covering on the ends of bones which forms a low friction surface for joint motion to occur.

Ibuprofen

A non-steroidal anti-inflammatory medication (or NSAID) which is used in the treatment of injuries to decrease pain and inflammation.

Ice pack

A flexible sack filled with crushed ice and applied to an injured body part to assist with the reduction of pain, swelling, and inflammation.

Ice massage

The use of a piece of solid ice rubbed directly on the skin for 8-10 minutes to achieve a reduction of pain, swelling, and inflammation.

Impingement syndrome

A painful inflammatory condition of the shoulder in which the tendons and bursa are injured by repeated pinching between bony structures during repetitive use of the upper arm. This is brought on by abnormal joint shape, poor muscle tone, or tight ligaments and joint capsule.

Inflammation

The normal cascade of cellular events triggered by traumatic or overuse injury. This process is the body's first response to injury and initiates the healing process.

Instability

A term used to describe the loss of the normal stability in a joint as a result of internal structural damage. This may also result from weakness of the muscles which cross that joint.

Internal rotation

A term used to describe motion of a bone or limb towards the midline of the body.

Intervertebral foramen

The opening formed between to vertebrae where the nerve root exits the spinal column. Lateral Stenosis is a condition which involves a narrowing of this opening placing abnormal pressure on the nerve root and leading to leg pain, numbness, or tingling.

Inversion ankle sprain

An ankle injury which results from the foot rolling inwards under the ankle and subsequent sprain injury to the ligaments that support the outside of the ankle.

Iontophoresis

The use of electrical current to drive electrically charged medications through the skin into inflamed ligaments, tendons, or other soft tissues.

Isometric contraction

The contraction of a muscle without any motion occurring.

Joint accessory motions

The additional gliding motion required in joint during bending or straightening. This motion can be improved with the application of joint mobilization techniques applied by a Physical Therapist.

Joint Capsule

A thin ligament material which surrounds each joint and functions to hold the bones together while also limiting excessive joint range of motion.

Kinematics

The description of joint motion using physical mechanics to help understand forces developed across a joint.

LCL(Lateral Collateral Ligament)

A ligament running vertically across the outside of the knee joint which functions to restrict excessive knee varus (bow legged), knee hyperextension, and lower leg internal rotation.

Lateral Epicondyle

A bony prominence on the outside of the elbow to which the Extensor Carpi Radialis Brevis is attached

Lateral epicondylitis

Inflammation and pain in the Extensor Carpi Radialis Brevis tendon where it attaches to the lateral epicondyle.

Lateral Meniscus

A half moon shaped cartilage located in the outer aspect of the knee joint. It functions to increase the congruency between the flat Tibia and curved Femur, absorb shock, and fight friction.

Lateral Stenosis

A narrowing of the space where nerve roots exit the spinal cord resulting in compression of those roots with corresponding leg symptoms.

Ligament

A soft tissue structure composed of dense fibers which attaches one bone to another and to limit the amount of motion available to the joint.

Lumbar corset

A wide band of fabric that can be wrapped around the circumference of the trunk to help provide a stabilizing effect to the low back, retain heat, and restrict excessive trunk motion.

Lumbar Disc

Found between each of the vertebral bones of the spine and is composed of the Annulus Fibrosus on the outside and the Nucleus Pulpous on the inside. The disc functions as an interconnection between bones, a shock absorber, and creates a flexible joint.

Lumbar disc herniation

The condition of a lumbar disc when some of the Annular rings become torn allowing the migration of the inner Nucleus Pulposus material backwards creating a bulge in the outer surface of the disc.

Lumbar lordosis

The backwards curve seen in the low back when viewed from the side. The amount of curvature can be described as excessive, balanced, or flat influenced by joint tightness or weak abdominals.

Manual therapy

This is the application of hands on therapeutic techniques for the mobilization of joints, muscles, and tendons. This is beneficial in the restoration normal joint accessory motions and to diminish abnormal muscle tone.

MCL (Medial Collateral Ligament)

The ligament found running vertically across the medial or inner aspect, of the knee joint. It is frequently sprained during twisting injuries of the knee.

Medial Epicondyle

A bony prominence on the inner aspect of the elbow to which the common flexor tendon is attached.

Medial Epicondylitis
  A condition of pain and inflammation of the common flexor tendon at its insertion on the Medial Epicondyle.

Medial Meniscus
  A quarter moon shaped piece of fibro-cartilage located between the Femur and the Tibia in the knee joint. It functions to provide improved congruency, to absorb shock, and reduce friction. It is frequently torn with twisting injuries of the knee.

MRI (Magnetic Resonance Imaging)
  A diagnostic machine that uses powerful magnets to create images of the body. Magnetic energy forces a quick flipping motion in water molecules which then emit a radio signal read by the machine.

Muscle
  This is the only soft tissue in the body which is capable of actively shortening or lengthening itself. Muscle contraction results in the production of forceful motion of a limb.

Musculoskeletal
  A term used to describe the entirety of the bony skeleton, ligaments, muscles, and tendons.

Nerve endings
  A general term used to describe the many types of microscopic sensory organs distributed throughout the body which are capable of detecting touch, pressure, heat, cold, vibration, and joint position.

Nerve Root
  The peripheral nerve which exits off the spinal cord through an opening between two vertebrae.

Neutral spine
  A term used to describe a position of the low back which is in a balanced posture and produces the least amount of pain. This position is individual to each spine and can be found by tilting the pelvis forward and backward until maximum comfort is detected.

Nucleus Pulposus
  A gelatinous fluid found in the center of spinal discs.

Palpation
  The act of using the hand to touch the body in order to determine the tactile quality of an injured soft tissue.

Paraspinal Muscle
  A muscle group which runs up and down each side of the spine and responsible for pulling the spine up from a forward bent position.

Pec
  An abbreviation for the Pectoralis muscles found in the chest or breast area.

Peripheral nervous system
  The general term used to describe all of the nerves outside of the central nervous system. The central nervous system includes the brain and the spinal cord.

Phonophoresis
  The use of ultrasound to physically push anti-inflammatory medications through the skin into inflamed tendons, ligaments, or other soft tissues.

PRICE
  An acronym used to describe first aide treatment techniques applied following injury.
  P= Protection, **R**= Rest, **I**= Ice, **C**= Compression, **E**= Elevation

PCL (Posterior Cruciate ligament)
A ligament located deep in the middle of the knee which helps restrict backward motion of the Tibia under the Femur, Tibial internal rotation, and hyperextension of the knee.

Posterior Talo-Fibular Ligament
A ligament which supports the outer aspect of the ankle and is commonly injured in a severe inversion ankle sprain.

Posture
The general term used to describe how body segments are aligned relative to one another.

Pronator Teres
A muscle in the forearm which functions to produce an inward twisting motion of the forearm resulting in a palm down position.

Prostaglandins
A molecular substance produced in the inflammation process which can create pain.

Protracted
A term which describes the forward shrugging motion of the shoulder blades.

Proprioceptive feedback
The ability of the body to detect joint position and motion of a limb in space using special sensors built into joints, ligaments, and tendons. This system is important to good balance and prevention of injury. This system can be improved with exercise.

Quadriceps muscles
The large muscle mass on the front of the thigh composed of four separate muscles. Contraction of this muscle group results in straightening of the knee joint.

Range of motion
A term used to describe the available motion a given joint is capable of moving through. It can also be used to describe any exercise activity designed to improve flexibility.

Referred Pain
Pain that is generated from an injury or illness in one part of the body, but that is sensed in a different location.

Repetitive motion injuries
Injury that results from repetitive overuse of a limb.

Retracted
A term which describes the backward shrugging motion of the shoulder blades.

Rest
An absence of activity.

Rotator cuff
A group of four small muscles which surround the shoulder joint and acts to center the ball of the shoulder in the middle of the joint socket.

Sacrum
A wedge shaped bone in the pelvis that forms the foundation for the lumbar spine.

Scapula
The shoulder blade bone commonly referred to as the "chicken wing".

Scar tissue
A type of connective tissue produced by the body during the healing process to initiate the repair of an injury.

Shoulder abduction
A term used to describe the direction of motion seen when lifting the arm out away from ones side.

Shoulder flexion
A term used to describe the direction of motion seen when lifting the arm up in front.

Soft tissues
A general term used to describe any connective body tissue which is soft and pliable.

Supraspinatus

One of four rotator cuff muscles crossing the top of the shoulder joint and is most frequently torn in a rotator cuff tear.

Spasm

The term used to describe the painful involuntary contraction of a muscle in response to injury or underlying joint pain.

Spinal cord

The bundle of nerve tissue which extends down from the brain through the center of the spine and carries nerve impulses both up and down from the brain.

Sprain

The term used to describe a sudden traumatic injury with resulting partial or complete tearing of ligaments.

Strain

The term used to describe a sudden traumatic injury with resulting partial or complete tearing of muscle tissue.

Strengthening

The process of improving muscle force development and size through the implementation of resistance exercises.

Stretching

The process of elongating muscle and improving joint flexibility through the application of a prolonged stretch at end range motion.

Subtalar Joint

The joint in the lower ankle which allows the foot to tilt in or out while walking as it adapts to side slopes and uneven terrain.

Synovial fluid

A fluid found inside of a joint which is produced by the synovial membrane lining the inside of a joint. It is responsible for assisting in lubrication and nutrition to the joint cartilage.

Talus

A small bone found in the center of the ankle joint.

Tendon

A bundle of dense parallel fibers attached to each end of a muscle and provides an attachment to bone. The tendon or its surrounding sheath is frequently the site of inflammation.

Tennis elbow

A term used to describe pain and inflammation of the tendon attached to the outside of the elbow. The medical term for this condition is Lateral Epicondylitis.

Theraband®

A brand named elastic rubber band material that is commonly used by physical therapists for administering home strengthening exercises.

Tendonitis

A term used to describe inflammation of a tendon.

Tibia

The larger of two parallel bones in the lower leg which is responsible for carrying most of the weight bearing forces through the lower leg to the ankle.

Tibial Plateau

A flat bony surface formed by the upper end of the Tibia bone which also forms the lower half of the knee joint.

Transverse Friction Massage

A massage technique where a perpendicular massage force is applied to deep structures by grabbing the skin with the finger tips and moving it back and forth quickly over the deeper tissues. Depth of pressure is increased as pain allows. This is commonly used to restore painfree function to injured ligaments and tendons.

Traumatic Injury

The sudden application of an external force which results in injury.

Ultrasound

A machine that emits high frequency sound energy which creates a heating effect in deep soft tissues. It is frequently used to improve circulation and reduce inflammation.

Valgus

A description of joint posture in which the lower segment is angled outward and the joint itself is angled inward (i.e. knocked knee = valgus).

Varus

A description of joint posture in which the lower segment is angled inward and the joint itself is angled outward (i.e. bow legged knee = varus).

Vertebra

Any one of 33 bones which makes up the spinal column.

Visceral

A term relating to internal organs or internal body cavity.

Warm-up effect

The decrease of pain experienced after several minutes of performing an activity. This is a good indication that inflammation is present.

Waiters Tip Stretch

A term used to describe a stretching position for the extensor muscles of the forearm. The position involves a straight elbow, internally rotated arm, and wrist bent to a palm up position which looks like a waiter accepting a tip behind his back

Winging scapula

A position of the scapula away from the rib cage so that a space forms between it and the trunk when viewed from behind. This can be the result of weakness in the muscles that support the scapula, or from a nerve injury.

Wrist Extension

The wrist motion which involves the backward bending of the hand with the palm is facing forward (i.e. wrist position needed to perform a push up with palms on the floor.)

Wrist Flexion

The wrist motion which is viewed as the wrist bends down and the palm is facing backwards.

Wrist Pronation/Supination

The wrist motion observed when the elbow is bent to 90 degrees and the hand is moved from a palm down position (pronation) to a palm up position (supination).